Baby-Led Weaning
for Busy Parents

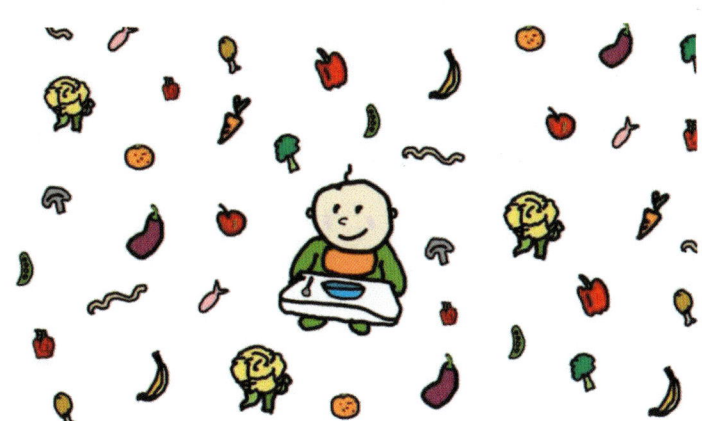

by

OLIVIA WITHALL

Copyright © Olivia Withall 2017
Photographs © Hannah Steenkamp and Olivia Withall 2017
Illustrations © Serena Wong 2017

Olivia Withall asserts her right to be identified as the author of this work in accordance with the Copyright, Designs and Patents Act 1988.

All rights reserved. No part of this publication may be reproduced, stored in a retrieval system, or transmitted in any form or by any means, electronic, mechanical, photocopying, recording or otherwise, without the prior permission of the copyright owner.

The information in this book has been compiled by way of general guidance in relation to the specific subjects addressed, but is not a substitute and not to be relied on for medical, healthcare, pharmaceutical or other professional advice on specific circumstances and in specific locations. Parents are advised to consult their health visitor, general practitioner or other relevant healthcare practitioner if they are concerned about their baby's health or development and before changing, stopping or starting any medical treatment. So far as the author is aware the information given is correct and up to date as at July 2017. Practice, laws, regulations and recommendations all change, and the reader should obtain up-to-date professional advice on any such issues. The author and publishers disclaim, as far as the law allows, any liability arising directly or indirectly from the use, or misuse, of the information contained in this book.

Copyright © 2017 Olivia Withall

All rights reserved.

ISBN: 9781521833377

DEDICATION

*I dedicate this book to my loving
and supportive husband, James,
and my gorgeous twins, Ace and Eve.*

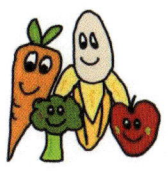

Baby-Led Weaning for Busy Parents
by Olivia Withall

CONTENTS

		Page
1	An Introduction to Baby-Led Weaning	1
2	Food for Teething	8
3	Basic Recipes	9
4	First Favourites	15
5	First Favourites: Recipes	16
6	Family Recipes	37
7	Snacks	64
8	Drinks	73
9	Weaning Diary	76
10	Daily Menu	79
11	Ace & Eve's Food Diary	81

ACKNOWLEDGMENTS

I would like to take this opportunity to thank my close friends in motherhood: Nicola Hatch-Lighterness and Hannah Steenkamp for helping me complete this book.

Edited by: **Nicola Hatch-Lighterness**
http://allthingsspliced.co.uk
https://www.facebook.com/AllThingsSpliced/

Photos edited by: **Hannah Steenkamp**
www.munchkinsphotography.co.uk
https://www.facebook.com/munchkinsfamilyphotography/

Thanks also go to my best friend and food tester, **Clare Mann** and my sister, Serena Wong, who drew the lovely cartoons included in this book.

Illustrations by: **Serena Wong**
https://pathofhappinessblog.com/
https://www.facebook.com/PathOfHappinessBlog/

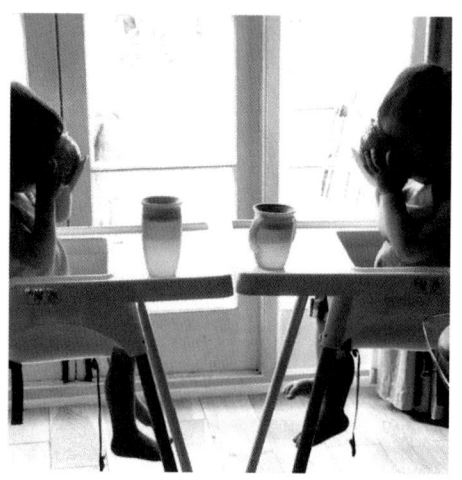

-♦♦- INTRODUCTION -♦♦-

Our Journey

I first heard about baby led weaning from my close friend, Hannah, when I was about to wean my twins at 6 months old. I saw how well her son was doing (he is 3 months older than the twins) and it appealed to me as it would give my kids a balanced diet but they could learn about new textures and flavours at the same time. I noticed that they tended to eat better if we are all sat at the table together and family mealtimes was something I wanted to encourage. I have always enjoyed cooking and felt passionate about knowing exactly what goes into the food that my children are eating. I'm not a super organic mother by any means, but I do like to know that their food is free from unnecessary preservatives and additives. By cooking meals from scratch I know exactly what is going into their food but also get a sense of satisfaction when they really love something (although of course there are times when I despair as they just aren't in the mood to eat and would rather play!).

The aim of this book is not to lecture others on how they should wean, but to give an overview of baby led weaning and share some of our favourite recipes with other busy parents. I used to spend hours dicing vegetables to make ratatouille (one of their favourites!) but I have now realised that a food processor, freezer or slow cooker can save so much time and effort and also that in the modern age there are lots of convenient options sold in supermarkets to help busy people spend less time prepping in the kitchen and more time eating delicious food and spending time with friends and family!

When can I start baby led weaning?

The UK Department of Health has recommended that babies will generally be ready for weaning at 6 months old as before this their digestive and immune systems aren't developed enough to manage solids (there are obviously some exceptions to this rule due to medical reasons).

As a parent you do tend to panic that your child is not getting enough nutrients when you start weaning, but it is helpful to remember that they will still be getting their nutrients from their milk feeds. When you start baby led weaning it is all about your child experiencing new flavours and textures more than eating for sustenance. Weaning is also a gradual process because it will take your child's body time to learn to digest solid food. Try not to worry too much if they don't eat much at the beginning as they will increase their portion sizes and naturally drop milk feeds when they feel ready.

For baby led weaning your baby should be able to do the following:

- Sit up without support
- Be proficient at grabbing toys etc.
- Make chewing or gnawing movements or try to grab food from your plate

What are the benefits of baby led weaning?

- Baby can be included in family mealtimes and doesn't have to eat separately
- Baby will be able to feed him/herself and learn what to do by watching what others are doing at the table
- Baby will decide how much to eat and learn to know their limits
- Baby will learn how to handle different shapes and textures of food
- Helps Baby to develop their coordination and dexterity
- Baby is less likely to be a picky eater as there isn't pressure on them to eat, which builds their confidence when trying new things

How often do I need to feed my child when starting BLW?

All families are different and have varying routines. There are a number of ways that you can start introducing solids. Some parents prefer to offer snacks throughout the day as 'tasters' for their children until they build up their appetite while others would rather offer meals. Our personal approach was to start with snacks such as pieces of fruit, houmous on toast etc. to grab their interest. After about two weeks we decided to offer them breakfast on a regular basis. This would usually involve yoghurt or porridge but sometimes toast or pikelets (flat crumpets) with unsalted or nut butter. As the twins started eating larger portions and becoming more enthusiastic I started to introduce lunch and eventually dinner. This whole process took a few months. A relatively simple approach could be to start with a meal that you feel would fit in with your family routine. Perhaps mornings are fraught and hectic as you're all trying to get to work or get other kids ready for school, so you could start offering lunch on a regular basis, or failing that dinner each evening.

Offering food should be a fun experience for your baby, so although you may feel anxious that they're not eating a lot try to remember that it is all about playing with colours, textures and flavours. The more laid back you appear (even if you are a nervous wreck inside) the more they will find enjoyment in trying new foods. When first starting out it is a good idea to choose a time when your little one isn't hungry or tired as they will be more likely to cooperate.

How do I know when my baby has finished eating?

You will soon learn their cues and be able to determine when your baby has finished eating. A few common signs are when they:

- Look around the room and seem disinterested.
- Start throwing their food around or onto the floor (rather than accidentally dropping it).
- Push their food away.
- Clamp their mouths shut!

The Gag Reflex

When starting to wean, a major worry for parents is that their little one will choke on solid food that hasn't been pureed. However, there has been research which indicates that although babies may seem as if they are choking it is in fact their gag reflex coming into play. The gag reflex in babies is a lot more sensitive compared to that of adults and is triggered further forward in the mouth. This means that when food goes too far back in the throat the baby will gag/retch and push the food forward to prevent it from entering their throat and airway (therefore avoiding choking). Gagging is a way that your baby to learns to eat safely as they teach themselves not to overfill their mouths or attempt to swallow before they have properly chewed the solid food.

It can be unnerving to watch your baby gagging and at first you might be scared that they are choking, but another way to reduce this is to ensure that your child is sitting up straight and in a supported position so that the food will fall forwards and out of their mouth should they gag (rather than back into their throat if they are in a reclined or laid back position).

The idea of baby led weaning is that your baby will feed themselves so they will control how much and how often food enters their mouth. This means that they will not only develop their motor skills but also be able to take their time to control the amount and regularity of each mouthful. If they are not ready to use cutlery you can always load a spoon up for them and leave it resting on their bowl/plate/table for them to pick up and feed themselves (or place it into their hand). This approach means that they are still in control of each mouthful and are less likely to choke as they aren't having food placed in their mouths before they are ready. Some babies only gag a few times when starting to wean whereas it takes others a little longer to get used to their gagging point. However, it is important to remember that your baby should never be left alone with food and should always be supervised.

My husband and I did read up on the gag reflex before weaning the twins, but as many other parents have done we also went on a baby and infant first aid course for peace of mind. You will be taught what to do in the event of real choking and also how to recognise it; actual choking is a silent occurrence whereas your baby will make some sort of noise if they are gagging/retching.

Foods to Avoid

There are a few ingredients that you need to be wary of when cooking baby led meals. However, as long as you have a general awareness it should be relatively easy to tailor your meals to accommodate this.

> **Salt** – when babies start weaning, their kidneys are unable to cope with large amounts of salt due to their immaturity, so it is best to avoid it as much as possible. If you like salt in your food then you could try cooking the meal without it and adding it to the adult portions at the end. However, I have found that we haven't really missed salt as we use a lot of herbs and spices which give each meal a stronger flavour. You may also want to be aware of hidden salts in ready made meals and sauces from the supermarket by taking a quick glance at the label (Daily Sodium Limits: Child aged 6-12 months = 1g of salt or 0.4g (400mg) of sodium, Child aged 1-2 years = 2g of salt or 0.8g (800mg) of sodium). Another thing to remember is that some foods (bacon, smoked fish, some cheeses etc.) contain natural salts so it is also good to use these sparingly if you are unable to avoid them.

> **Sugar** – research has shown that if you avoid giving children a sugary diet in their early years they will be less likely to have a sweet tooth when they are older. Once again, there are often hidden sugars in mass produced foods such as sauces, cereals, tinned fruit, baked beans, flavoured yoghurts etc. Fruit contains natural sugars and can be used as a sweetener in desserts. Additionally, you may wish to be careful when buying 'sugar free' products as they can contain artificial/chemical sweeteners instead.

Personally, I believe in living with a general awareness of the ingredients contained in pre-packaged food and think twice when buying them as even meals labelled as 'low fat' have a huge amount of processed ingredients as well as salt, sugar, additives etc. to enhance the flavour and texture of the food. As with all things in life, I think that "everything in moderation" is a good way to approach both salt and sugar – a little now and then is fine!

- **High-fibre foods** – bran and high-fibre cereals can interfere with the absorption of iron and other nutrients so are not suitable for babies.

- **Honey** – babies should not be given honey until they are one year old as although very rare, it can be the source of an infection called botulism.

Foods to be careful of

- **Grapes and cherry tomatoes** – make sure that these are halved (or even better, quartered) lengthways to avoid accidental choking.

- **Citrus fruits** – be careful of the pith/white bits as this is hard for babies to chew and can cause gagging/choking.

- **Whole nuts** – these are not suitable for babies as they may cause choking.

- **Hard fruits** (such as apples etc.) – offer these in large pieces or whole so that baby can bite into them.

- **Runny eggs** – eggs often contain salmonella. The current advice is for babies to only eat runny eggs if they have the lion mark on them, as the hens producing them have been vaccinated against salmonella. Fully cooked eggs with a firm yolk are fine, but approach food that may contain raw eggs (such as homemade mayonnaise) with caution.

Allergies

If there is a history of food allergies in your family then it has been advised that parents introduce new foods slowly and allow at least three days between foods that may be likely to cause an allergic reaction. Common foods that cause allergies are:

- Cow's milk/Lactose
- Nuts
- Wheat and Gluten
- Seafood
- Strawberries

Drinks to Avoid

Babies can have fresh tap water from 6 months of age. Breast and formula milk will still be their main source of nutrients and babies should never be given caffeinated or very sugary drinks. Cow's milk shouldn't be introduced until your baby is 1 year old but is fine to use in cooking or cereal, provided that it has been pasteurised (in fact, using it in cereal and cooking is a good way for babies to get used to both digesting it and the taste). Pure fruit juice is fine in small quantities or just a tiny amount in water, but large amounts of juice shouldn't be given as although it is free from additives it contains a lot of sugar.

Early Days

In the early days of weaning we kept a food diary. This is not necessary at all (unless your baby has an intolerance or allergy, perhaps), but we liked to refer to it to see what foods the kids enjoyed eating and others that they were not keen on. It is recommended that if your child dislikes a certain food it should be offered to them more than once (about 6 times) so that they can get used to the flavour and feel of it in their mouth before officially deciding they don't like something.

We were very surprised that the twins were able to use spoons (which we helped them load) from day one as we had expected them to miss their mouths and create a mess! We would always offer them cutlery and they got on well with it but were equally happy to use their hands. However, at about 1 year old (the twins are now 2 and a half) my son decided he didn't like his cutlery anymore and would use his hands! This is all fine as he likes to feel the texture of the foods he is eating and we sometimes joke that he is a food critic in the making as he seems to be able to tell how ripe/sweet fruit is just by holding it in his hands first!

This is an example of our weaning diary (the original is a lot more rudimentary and scribbled into a notebook!) and a sample page is included at the end of the book:

Date	Food	Like	Unsure	Dislike
Monday 2 May	Greek yoghurt with stewed apple	✓		

Tidy House, Tidy Mind?

When the babies first started on solids we would feed them in the kitchen so that the mess could be mopped or swept up. It is interesting that people have different approaches to this; I would be frantically scrubbing all the clumps of food up with a wet cloth whereas my husband would wait for it to dry a little and hoover it all up! If you are worried about the mess then it could be helpful to put an old plastic tablecloth or mat on the floor which can easily be cleaned to avoid damaging the floor in your home! Alternatively, a good investment (in addition to your trusty dustpan and brush) is a steam mop which is good at removing grime and bits of food/sauce which have stuck to the floor. In addition, suction bowls are also useful as they prevent your baby from tipping or throwing their food everywhere.

What Bib Should My Baby Wear?

There are many weaning bibs on the market, but the type that you opt for generally depends on yourself and your child. There are plastic ones with a pocket at the bottom to catch food, fabric ones and also plastic/fabric apron-style bibs.

Primarily I tried the harder plastic bibs with the pocket on the twins which worked for a while as they were only eating large finger foods, but it soon got messy when they got stuck into their porridge! I then thought that a fully plastic apron-style bib would work well as it would keep their clothes clean and dry. Unfortunately, this also didn't go entirely to plan as the food would just slide down the bib and onto their laps, feet and the floor! Eventually, we stumbled upon fabric apron bibs with a plastic backing. They soon became a firm favourite as they soak up any wet food, but the plastic forms a protective layer which doesn't allow it to permeate through the bib onto their clothing. However, now that the twins are older and relatively neat with their eating we have gone back to the original plastic pocket bib!

To Batch or not to Batch?

I am a big fan of batch cooking and freezing as it means that there is always food to hand if we are late home from somewhere and need a quick ready meal or if the twins are being babysat and need to be given a healthy meal. However, I know that not everyone has a large freezer so batch cooking may not be suitable for those families. Nevertheless, baby led weaning recipes are useful as they are meals that the whole family can enjoy together so if there are any leftovers they can always go into the fridge ready to be eaten (or rehashed into another meal!) the next day. Alternatively, if you do have freezer space you can always portion up leftovers and keep them in the freezer for easy use as and when you need them.

FOOD FOR TEETHING

There are some foods that we found were helpful in times of teething. Yes, some of them are hard in texture, but the babies would like the cool feeling of them against their gums and gnaw on them rather than eat them as a meal:

- Cucumber sticks
- Fruit sticks (such as melon, mango, pineapple)
- Greek or Natural Yoghurt (sweetened with crushed berries or stewed apple, peach or pear)
- Frozen banana (thawed a little or slightly mashed)
- Fruit juice lollies (I would use watered down fruit juice to reduce the amount of sugar consumed)
- Milk lollies
- Ready made formula or expressed breast milk straight from the fridge

-♦♦- BASIC RECIPES -♦♦-

These are things that I make regularly for quick use in a variety of meals (*they can also be frozen, which is handy!*).

Stewed Fruit

Good fruits to use are apples, pears, peaches, plums, nectarines.

Method:

1. Dice your fruit and place them in a small pan over a medium heat.
2. Add a splash of water and cook for 5 to 10 minutes until the fruit has softened and broken down. Add a little more water if needed.
3. If you wish, mush the mixture slightly but be sure to leave small chunks in it to give texture/something for baby to gum down on.

- ❖ Use the stewed fruit to sweeten: porridge, yoghurts, spread on toast or bread as a jam, in cakes or biscuits instead of sugar.
- ❖ Can be stored in the fridge for up to a week or in small pots in the freezer for 2 months.

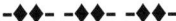

Alternative twist – you can also stew berries which shouldn't need cutting as they will naturally break down. However, if you are using large strawberries then perhaps dice them to make the cooking time quicker. You could buy mixed fruit (smoothie mixes) from the frozen aisle at the supermarket and try stewing those to make interesting flavour combinations.

Vegetable Stock

2 large white onions

3 sticks of celery

3 large carrots

1 clove of garlic

1 bay leaf

A pinch of black pepper

1.5 litres of boiling water

Method:

1. Dice or grate all of your vegetables and place to one side.
2. Heat a little oil in a pot over a medium heat.
3. Add the vegetables to the pot and fry gently until slightly softened (or at least until the onions have softened).
4. Add the bay leaf and 1.5 litres of boiling water from the kettle.
5. Simmer for 20 to 30 minutes.
6. Strain the stock and either use straight away or cool and refrigerate/freeze ready for use.

Storage – can be stored in the fridge for a couple of days or frozen in ice cube trays or plastic tubs for up to 2 months.

Time Boost – use a food processor to chop your vegetables or you can buy pre-chopped veg at the supermarket to save you some effort!

Effort Saver - after softening the onion, place all of the vegetables into a slow cooker with the water and leave to simmer for a few hours.

Money Saver – you can use your old vegetable scraps from cooking other things to make this! Store them in a bag in the freezer as you go along and when the bag is full then use your veg scraps to make a delicious stock!

Alternative twist - add a little cornflour to some of the stock and vegetables to thicken and serve as a clear soup. Or try blending the stock and veg with a little cream or milk to create a simple but delicious vegetable soup! To make a thicker soup, blend with mashed potatoes. Alternatively, use the stock to make cous cous as it will give it a little flavour.

Pasta Sauce

1 large white onion

4 tomatoes, chopped

500g of Passata

1 bay leaf

2 sprigs of thyme

A pinch of ground black pepper (or 1/4 teaspoon cayenne pepper)

Method:
1. Peel and grate the onion before discarding any water that comes out of it.
2. Place it in a large pot and gently fry until golden.
3. Add the remaining ingredients and simmer over a medium heat for 30 - 40 minutes (or longer if you want a thicker, richer sauce), stirring occasionally and adding water if you prefer a thinner sauce.

Storage – can be stored in the fridge for a couple of days or frozen in portion sizes for up to 2 months.

Alternative Twist – you can try adding the following to your preference:
- Crushed garlic (fry with the onions until golden)
- Grated carrot or chopped red peppers (will give the sauce a sweeter taste)
- Chopped spinach or a tin of green lentils (this will boost the iron and protein levels)
- Herbs such as basil, oregano or rosemary
- Spices such as paprika

Time Boost – use a food processor to chop your onions and tomatoes. You can buy passata with garlic and herbs added from the supermarket.

Effort Saver – after frying the onions you can place all of this into a slow cooker and leave it to simmer for a few hours.

White Sauce

50g unsalted butter

50g plain flour

500ml whole milk

1 Bay leaf

A pinch of nutmeg

Method:
1. Melt the butter in a pan before adding the flour and nutmeg.
2. Mix together to form a roux and continue to cook over a medium heat for 2 minutes, stirring all the time.
3. Put the bay leaf into the pan and gradually add the milk (using a whisk will help to keep the sauce smooth) until the sauce thickens.
4. Remove the bay leaf before serving.

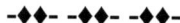

Storage – can be stored in the fridge for a couple of days or frozen in portion sizes for up to 2 months.

Alternative Twist – use this method to make a variety of sauces:
- Add a tiny bit of grated cheese to make cheese sauce (75g for babies)
- Add some Dijon or English mustard paste/powder to make a mustard sauce
- Add ground pepper to make a pepper sauce
- Fry some mushrooms in with the butter and flour before adding the milk to make mushroom sauce

Roasted Vegetable Mix

2 courgettes

1 large aubergine

1 large red onion

1 large white onion

1 red pepper, deseeded

4 cloves of garlic, crushed

A pinch of black pepper

2 tablespoons of olive oil

Method:
1. Set your oven to 200C/392F.
2. Dice all of the vegetables and place onto a baking tray.
3. Drizzle over the olive oil and mix it into the vegetables to make sure they are all covered. Season with the pepper.
4. Roast for 30-40 minutes until the vegetables have slightly caramelised, giving them a mix halfway through.

- ❖ Use in: ratatouille or to make pasta sauces (mix it into the recipe above!) or vegetable tarts (see recipes for these further on in the book). Alternatively, you can mix it in with cous cous for a delicious dish!

Storage – can be stored in the fridge for a couple of days or frozen in portion sizes for up to 2 months.

Time Boost – use a food processor to chop all of your vegetables!

-♦♦- FIRST FAVOURITES -♦♦-

Rather than pureeing food I decided to offer the twins 'soft foods' as part of their diet when we first started. A few simple ideas are:

- Greek yoghurt (plain or sweetened with stewed fruit)
- Houmous (with toast or pitta bread fingers)
- Porridge oats (sweetened with stewed fruit)
- Fruit
- Roasted vegetables (this was a good starting point as the veg is hard enough to grip, but soft enough to be mushed between gums)
- Cous cous (flavoured with no salt vegetable stock or roasted vegetables)
- Rice pudding (flavoured with vanilla or sweetened with stewed fruit)
- Pikelets (flat crumpets) or rice cakes (with 100% nut butters, such as almond, peanut or cashew or with unsalted butter)
- Pancakes (plain or sweetened with stewed fruit)
- Jacket Potatoes (with a little bit of cheese, tuna (tinned in spring water rather than brine), unsalted butter)

(The twins also liked toast, cucumber and melon to suck on!)

-♦♦- FIRST FAVOURITES: RECIPES -♦♦-

PORRIDGE

2 mins preparation
2-3 mins cooking

50g Rolled Oats (Scottish or Quaker)
300ml full fat milk

Method:

1. Put the oats and milk into a pan and mix well.

2. Bring to the boil and simmer for 2-3 minutes, stirring continuously.

3. Add more milk if you want a looser consistency.

4. Check the temperature and serve with stewed or chopped dried fruit for flavour and sweetness.

Time/Effort Boost - cook the porridge in your microwave on high for 2 minutes. Remove and add more milk if desired to make it looser but it will also cool the porridge down a little.

Fruit Fact - I found this a good way to get fruits into my babies when they hadn't been eating a lot of it or when they were clogged up and needed to loosen their bowels. Good dried fruit to use for this are prunes, dates, figs, raisins and apricots.

HOUMOUS

10 mins preparation time

200g/small tin of chickpeas
90g Natural or Greek yoghurt
Squeeze of lemon juice
A pinch of black pepper
1 teaspoon of olive oil

Method:

1. Place all of the ingredients into a blender and blend away until you reach your desired texture!

2. Serve as a dip or spread on toast.

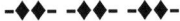

Alternative Twist – add red peppers, caramelised red onion, roasted garlic, herbs (like coriander etc.) or spices (such as paprika) to make different flavours! If you find your houmous too thin in texture then simply add in more chickpeas.

WHIPPED YOGHURT MOUSSE

10 mins preparation
2 hours setting time
Serves 4

150ml Greek yoghurt
150ml double cream

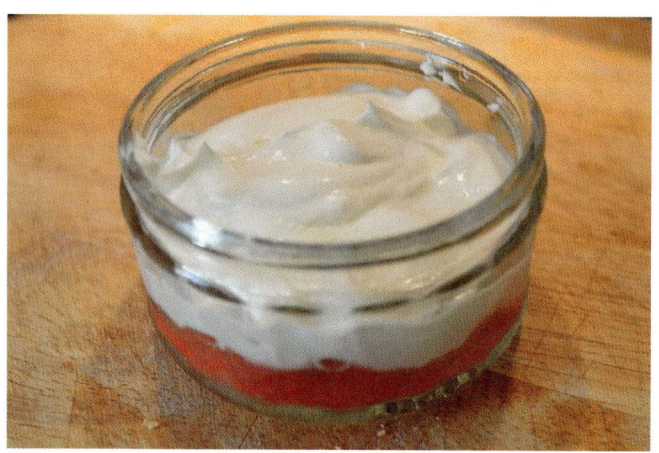

Method:

1. Put the double cream into a deep bowl and whip until it forms peaks.

2. Carefully fold in the yoghurt, a little at a time, making sure you don't knock too much air out of the cream.

3. Spoon the mixture into ramekins, cover with cling film and leave to set in the fridge for at least 2 hours.

4. Serve plain or with fresh/stewed fruit as a snack, dessert or treat!

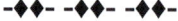

Alternative Twist - put stewed fruit at the bottom of the ramekin before adding the yoghurt mixture on top. Or perhaps you could try carefully folding some stewed fruit into the yoghurt mixture to make flavoured yoghurt. For children over 1 year old, a little drizzle of honey is delicious with this!

SUNDRIED TOMATO BUTTER

This delicious butter is great served on toast, crackers or rice/corn cakes!

3 mins preparation
10-15 mins cooking
2 hours setting
Makes 3 blocks

280g jar of sundried tomatoes
280ml double cream
A pinch of black pepper
A pinch of Italian seasoning (usually a mix of oregano and basil)

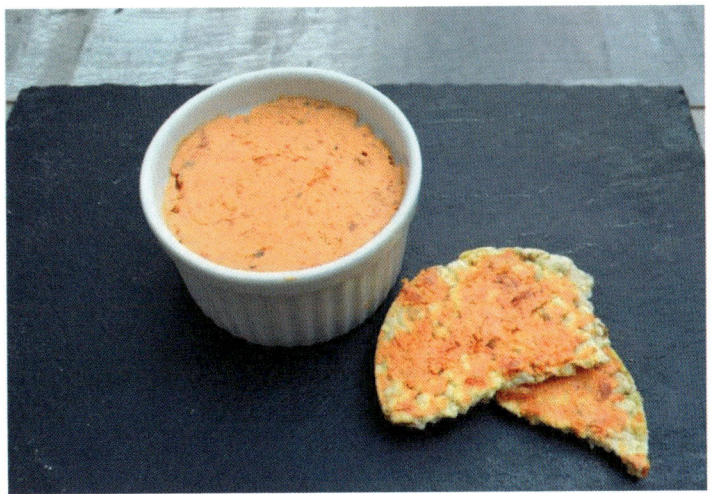

Method:

1. Remove the sundried tomatoes from the oil that they are preserved in and place on a kitchen towel. Press lightly to remove excess oil.

2. Place the sundried tomatoes into a blender or food processor along with the double cream.

3. Blend for 10-15 minutes until smooth (about halfway through the mixture will start to look wet and crumbly, continue blending past this).

4. Put the butter into ramekins and place in the fridge for at least 2 hours to set.

5. Serve!

Storage - store in the fridge or can be wrapped up tightly and kept in the freezer for up to 2 months.

Money Saver - remember to keep the oil that the sundried tomatoes were preserved in as it is great to use for cooking risottos or pasta dishes.

RICE PUDDING

5 mins preparation
35 mins cooking time
Serves 4

100g pudding rice
850ml full fat milk
1/2 large vanilla pod or 1 teaspoon vanilla extract

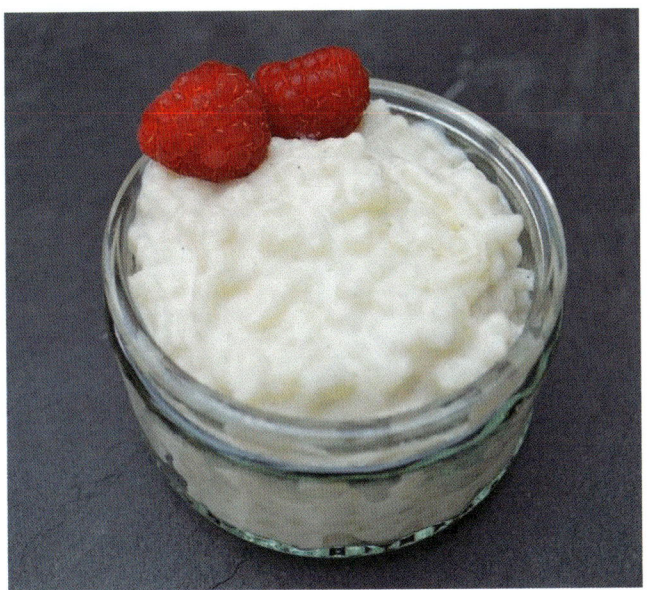

Method:

1. Split the vanilla pod in half and remove the seeds. Add the seeds and pod into the milk.

2. Put the pudding rice and milk into a non-stick saucepan over a medium heat. Bring it to the boil, stirring continuously.

3. Reduce the heat and gently simmer for 35 minutes, stirring all the time until the rice is soft.

4. Serve hot or cold as a delicious breakfast, snack or dessert!

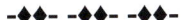

Alternative Twist - serve with stewed fruit to add sweetness and flavour or sprinkle a little nutmeg or cinnamon over the top!

Effort Boost - you can also cook this in the oven - heat your oven to 180C/356F and put all of the ingredients into an ovenproof dish, making sure it is mixed well. Bake in the centre of the oven for 30 minutes. Stir and return to the oven for another 60-90 minutes or until a lightly browned skin has formed on the surface of the pudding.

RATATOUILLE

15 mins preparation
30 mins cooking
Serves 4-6

1 large red onion
1 large aubergine
1 large red pepper
2 courgettes
4 tomatoes
400g tin of chopped tomatoes
1 teaspoon of oregano
Olive oil
A pinch of black pepper

Method:

1. Dice all of the vegetables to a suitable size for your child.
2. Heat a little olive oil in a pan over a medium heat and add the onion. Fry gently until softened.
3. Add all of the remaining ingredients and stir to ensure they are well mixed.
4. Simmer the ratatouille for 20 -30 minutes or until the tomatoes thicken to form a sauce, stirring occasionally. If the ratatouille looks too thick, then add a splash of water halfway through.
5. Serve with pasta, cous cous or bread.

Storage - can be kept in the fridge for a couple of days and reheated. Alternatively, the ratatouille can be divided in portions and frozen for up to 2 months.
Time Boost – use a food processor to dice all of your vegetables.
Effort Boost – after softening the onion, put all of the ingredients into a slow cooker and allow to simmer for a few hours. Alternatively, if you have any of the 'Roasted Vegetable Mix' from earlier in the book to hand, simply add this to a tin of tomatoes and 1 teaspoon of oregano and simmer until the sauce is thick.
Veggie Boost – add chopped spinach (you can get chopped frozen spinach too!), chickpeas or lentils to boost the iron and protein.
Alternative Twist – serve mixed with pasta and a tin of tuna (preserved in spring water rather than brine) for a delicious pasta dish!

EGG AND TOMATO SCRUMBLE

10 mins preparation
10 mins cooking
Serves 4

4 large eggs
1 teaspoon of sesame oil
1/3 of a teaspoon of white pepper
6 tomatoes, skinned and cut into wedges
1/2 a level teaspoon of sugar
3 spring onions, chopped

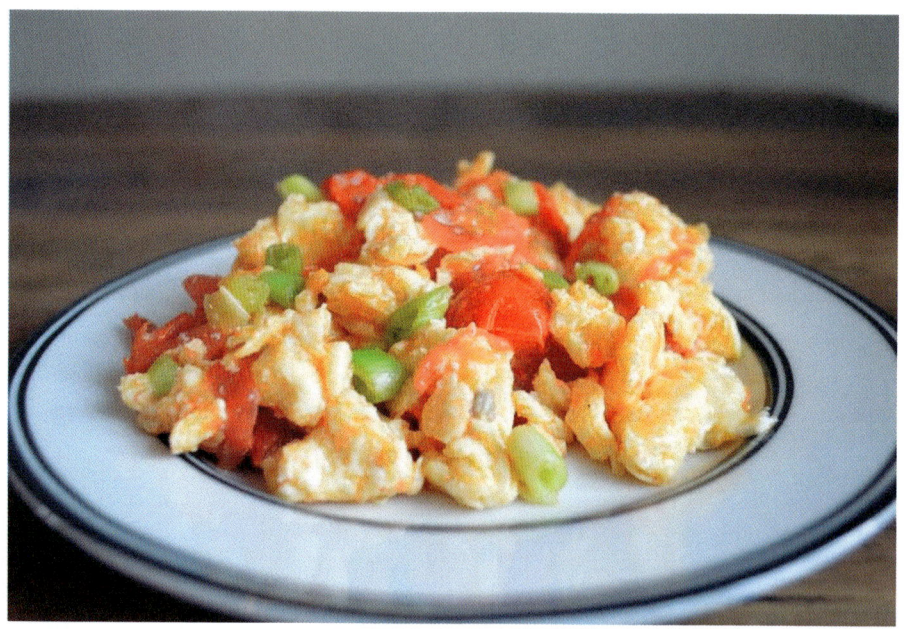

Method:

1. Beat the eggs in a bowl with the sesame oil and white pepper.

2. Heat a little oil in a pan over a medium heat and add the egg mixture. Scramble the eggs then place them in a bowl and set aside.

3. Add a little more oil to the pan and throw in the tomatoes and sugar. Fry them gently until the tomatoes have completely broken down, almost forming a sauce. Add little splashes of water into the pan if the tomatoes look like they are getting too dry or sticking to the sides.

4. Add the eggs back into the pan along with the chopped spring onions. Stir and mix everything together until the eggs are reheated.

5. Serve immediately with rice, on its own as a snack or with crunchy toast!

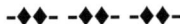

Vegan Twist – use a block of soft or firm tofu instead of the egg, it is just as delicious!

Time Boost – to remove the tomato skins, blanch the tomatoes in boiling water for 1 minute then shock them in a bowl of cold water. The skins should then come off easily.

LENTIL DAAL (CURRY)

10 mins preparation
15 mins cooking
Serves 4

150g red split lentils
3 medium/260g tomatoes
1 large onion
2 large cloves of garlic, crushed
2cm ginger, peeled and finely grated
1 teaspoon of cumin seeds
1/2 a teaspoon of black mustard seeds
1 teaspoon of ground turmeric
1 teaspoon of garam massala
1 teaspoon of dry coriander leaves
A pinch of black pepper
200ml boiling water

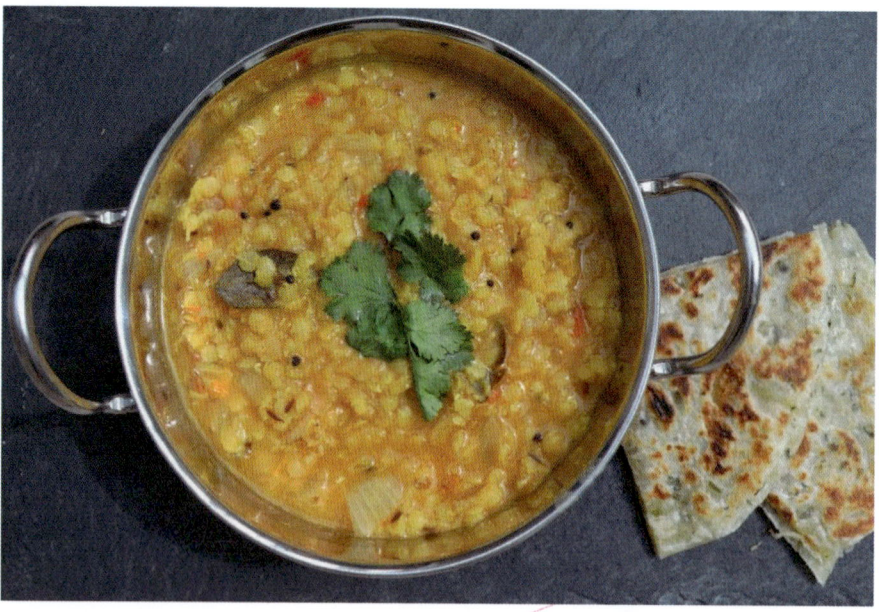

Method:

1. Rinse the lentils and place in a pan with enough boiling water to cover them. Boil for 10-15 minutes until cooked (they will become soft and puff up).

2. Meanwhile, dice your onion and tomatoes to a size that suits your baby.

3. Put a little oil in a pan and add the cumin and mustard seeds. Fry until fragrant and they start popping.

4. Add the onion, garlic and ginger and fry until golden.

5. Put the tomatoes and the rest of the spices into the pan and mix well.

6. Add 200ml of boiling water and cook for 5 minutes.

7. Drain the cooked lentils and add them to the tomato mixture. Stir well and cook for another 5 minutes (add more water if it looks a little dry - it should be a loose, soupy texture).

8. Serve with rice, naan bread or on its own!

Alternative Twist - if you put the daal in a blender you can turn it into a delicious lentil soup! Add a bit of coconut milk or sprinkle some fresh coriander on top if you want an alternative flavour. You can also slice shallots and fry until crispy before sprinkling on top or mixing in - this gives it a deeper, sweeter flavour.

Veggie Boost - try adding chopped spinach or a handful of peas to the daal. You can even add small bits of diced potato or carrots.

Time Boost - use a food processor to dice your onion and tomatoes or garlic. Alternatively, instead of dicing tomatoes, use half of a 400g tin of chopped tomatoes.

Storage – this can be frozen in portions for up to 2 months.

BEAN CHILLI

5 mins preparation
25 mins cooking
Serves 4-6

1 large red onion, diced to a suitable size for your child

1 red pepper, deseeded and diced to a suitable size for your child

400g tin of green, brown or black lentils

200g/small tin of red kidney beans (in water)

200g/small tin of chickpeas

400g tin of chopped tomatoes or 8 fresh tomatoes, diced to a suitable size for your child

1 tablespoon of olive oil

2 heaped teaspoons of cumin

1 teaspoon of smoked paprika

1/2 a teaspoon of cayenne pepper

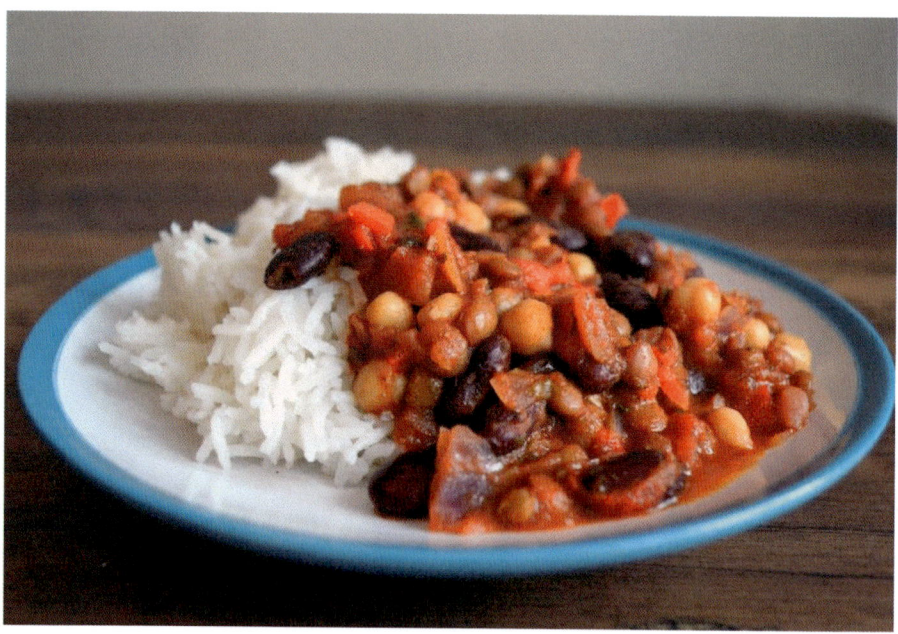

Method:

1. Heat the olive oil in a pan over a medium heat. Add the onion and fry until golden.

2. Add the red pepper and fry until softened.

3. Place all of the remaining ingredients into the pan and mix well.

4. Simmer for 20-25 minutes, stirring occasionally until the sauce thickens and the beans start to break down slightly.

5. Serve with rice, cous cous, pasta, sweet potato wedges or a jacket potato!

-♦♦- -♦♦- -♦♦-

Storage - can be kept in the fridge for a couple of days and reheated. Alternatively, the bean chilli can be divided in portions and frozen for up to 2 months.

Time Boost – use a food processor to dice your onion, red pepper and fresh tomatoes (if using).

Effort Boost – after softening the onion and pepper, put all of the ingredients into a slow cooker and allow to simmer for a few hours.

Veggie Boost – add in some chopped spinach to boost the iron content.

Alternative Twist – try adding some herbs (such as coriander). If you like a spicier bean chilli you could add some chilli powder or increase the amount of cayenne pepper. Add in beef mince after you have fried the onion to make a delicious chilli con carne. Alternatively, serve with homemade tortilla chips (recipe further on in the book) for a delicious snack.

CAULIFLOWER AND BROCCOLI CHEESE

10 mins preparation
20 mins cooking
Serves 4

350g cauliflower florets
350g broccoli florets
50g unsalted butter
50g plain flour
500ml whole milk
1 bay leaf
A pinch of nutmeg
100g cheese, grated

Method:

1. Set your oven to 200C/392F.

2. Wash the cauliflower and broccoli and place in a large pot.

3. Boil until tender (about 5-10 minutes) or as soft as your child can manage. Break the florets into smaller sizes if necessary for your child (but try not to mush it all up) and set aside.

4. Meanwhile, melt the butter in a large pot before adding the flour and nutmeg.

5. Mix everything together to form a roux and continue to cook over a medium heat for 2 minutes, stirring all the time.

6. Put the bay leaf into the pot and gradually add the milk (using a whisk will help to keep the sauce smooth) until the sauce thickens.

7. Add 75g of the cheese and mix into the sauce until melted.

8. Remove the bay leaf. Take the broccoli and cauliflower and mix well into the sauce.

9. Place into an ovenproof dish and sprinkle the remaining cheese over the top.

10. Cook in the oven for 15 minutes or until the cheese on top turns golden.

11. Serve and let your children use their hands!

-♦♦- -♦♦- -♦♦-

Storage – can be stored in the fridge for a couple of days or frozen in portion sizes for up to 2 months.

Time/Effort Boost – you can use ready made white sauce that you might already have in the freezer (see recipe at beginning of the book) and simply heat it up and add cheese to make the sauce. After making up the broccoli and cauliflower cheese you can even serve immediately rather than browning the top in the oven.

Alternative Twist – I often add cooked macaroni into the mix too! For older children you can also try adding a bit of diced ham. If you like a bit of a crunch, top with fresh breadcrumbs before putting it in the oven.

POTATO WEDGES

10 mins preparation
30-40 mins cooking
Serves 4-6

8 medium to large potatoes

2 teaspoons of cumin

1/2 teaspoon of cayenne pepper (optional)

1 teaspoon of dried coriander leaf

1 teaspoon of smoked paprika

1 tablespoon of tomato puree

2 tablespoons of oil

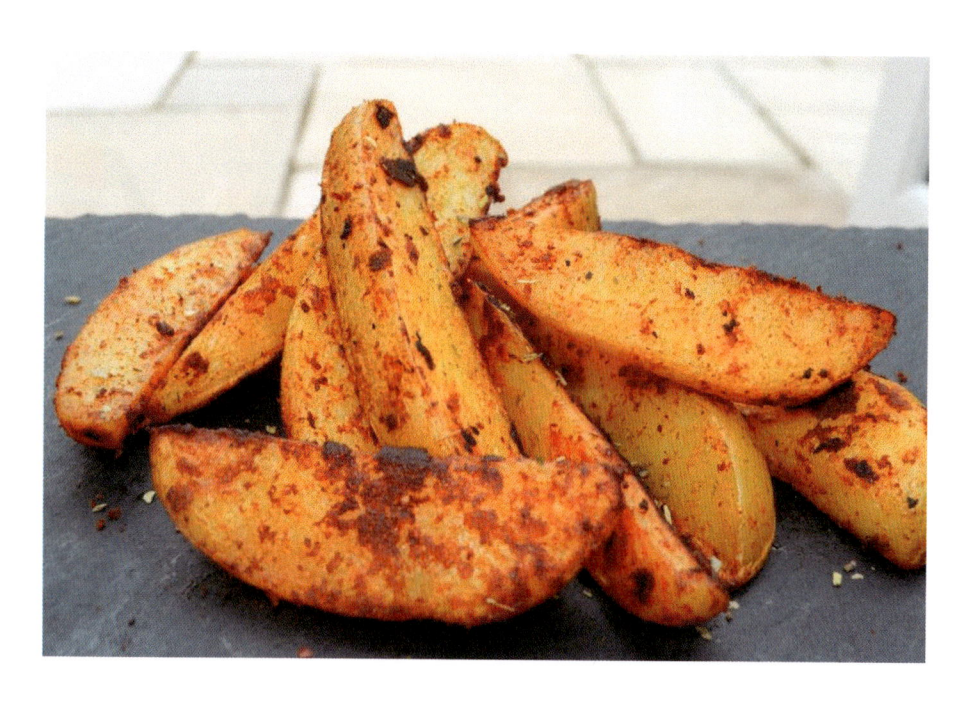

Method:

1. Set the oven to 200C/392F.
2. Scrub the potatoes until clean and cut them into wedges. Place the wedges onto a non-stick baking tin or tray.
3. Mix the remaining ingredients together to form a paste.
4. Pour the paste over the wedges and use your hands to make sure all of them are thoroughly covered in the spices.
5. Cook for 30-40 minutes until golden and cooked through.
6. Remove from the oven and serve as a delicious side dish or snack!

-♦♦- -♦♦- -♦♦-

Alternative Twist - try using sweet potato or adding your own favourite herbs/spices into the mix!

PAELLA

10 mins preparation
25 mins cooking
Serves 4-6

2 tablespoons of olive oil
1 large white onion, diced to a suitable size for your child
4 cloves of garlic, crushed
1 cup of white rice
1/4 teaspoon of saffron strands
400g/1 tin of chopped tomatoes
1 large red pepper, deseeded and sliced
2 cups vegetable stock (very low salt, found in most major supermarkets or use the recipe at the beginning of the book)
1 cup beans (kidney, cannellini or haricot work well)
1 cup frozen peas

Method:

1. Heat the olive oil in a pan over a medium heat and fry the onion and garlic for 3 minutes.
2. Add the rice and saffron and fry for another minute.
3. Throw in the tomatoes, pepper and beans and stir for 1 minute.
4. Add the vegetable stock and bring the mixture to the boil.
5. Reduce the heat, cover and simmer the paella for 10 minutes.
6. Check the paella and add a bit of water if needed.
7. Stir in the peas and cook until the peas are tender and the rice has absorbed any liquid.

-♦♦- -♦♦- -♦♦-

Alternative Twist - add cooked seafood, chicken or chorizo (be careful of the salt content in this) for extra flavour!

SWEETCORN FRITTERS

10 mins preparation
20 mins cooking
Makes 24

170g self raising flour

250ml milk

280g (or 1 large tin) of sweetcorn

1 red pepper, diced to a suitable size for your child

3 spring onions, chopped

1 teaspoon of paprika

A pinch of black pepper (or 1/2 teaspoon of cayenne pepper)

Oil for shallow frying

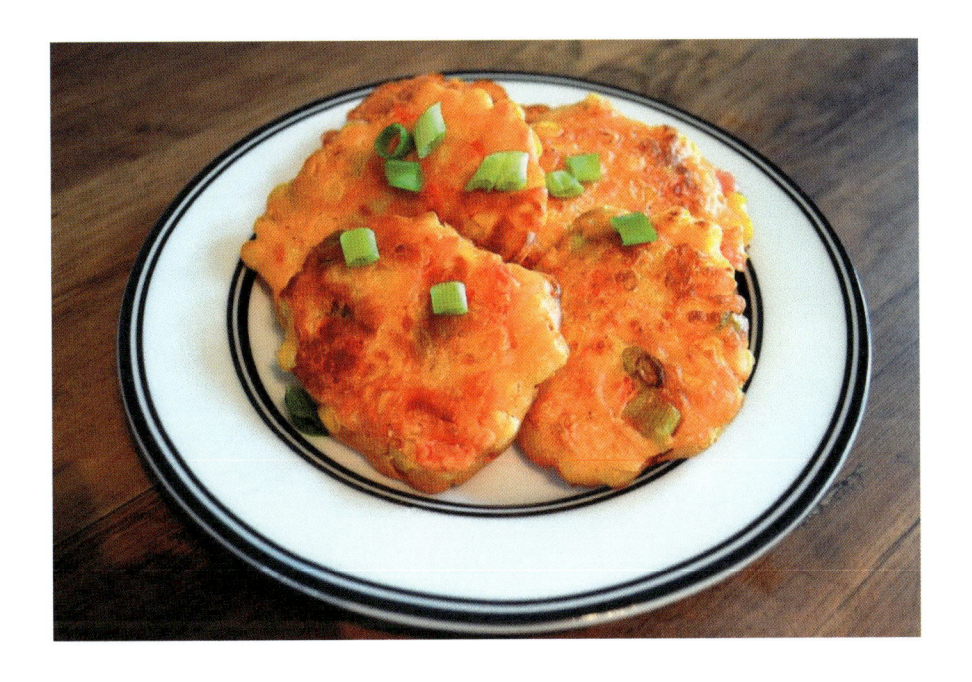

Method:

1. Put the self raising flour into a large mixing bowl and stir in the paprika and black pepper.
2. Gradually pour the milk into the flour mixture and whisk until smooth.
3. Add the sweetcorn, red pepper, spring onions and mix until covered by the batter.
4. Heat a little oil in a pan and once hot put heaped dessert spoonfuls of the mixture into the pan and flatten slightly.
5. Fry until golden then turn the fritters over and cook the other side.
6. Drain on kitchen paper and serve once slightly cooled!

-♦♦- -♦♦- -♦♦-

Storage – can be kept in the fridge for a couple of days and reheated or served cold as a snack. Alternatively, they can be frozen for up to 2 months and reheated in a pan directly from frozen.

Time Boost - if you're short of time you can substitute the sweetcorn and red pepper for a tin of sweetcorn with the peppers already added.

Veggie Boost - why not turn these into vegetable fritters by adding extra vegetables? Peas, mushrooms, courgette etc. work well!

Alternative Twist - try adding cooked fish or a can of drained tuna (in spring water) to make simple fishcakes. Or perhaps add small bits of ham or sausage for older children.

-♦♦- IT'S A FAMILY AFFAIR! -♦♦-

Now that your baby is well practised in eating solids they can have even more fun with food and family at the dinner table!

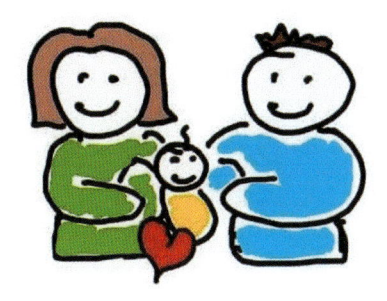

ROASTED VEGETABLE ORZO

15 mins preparation
40 mins cooking
Serves 4-6

Roasted Vegetable Mix

1 aubergine

2 large red onions

2 red peppers, deseeded

4 cloves of garlic, crushed

A pinch of black pepper

2 tablespoons of olive oil

Orzo and Dressing

220g orzo pasta

Juice of 1/2 a lemon

1 tablespoon of olive oil

A pinch of black pepper

6 fresh basil leaves, chopped or ripped

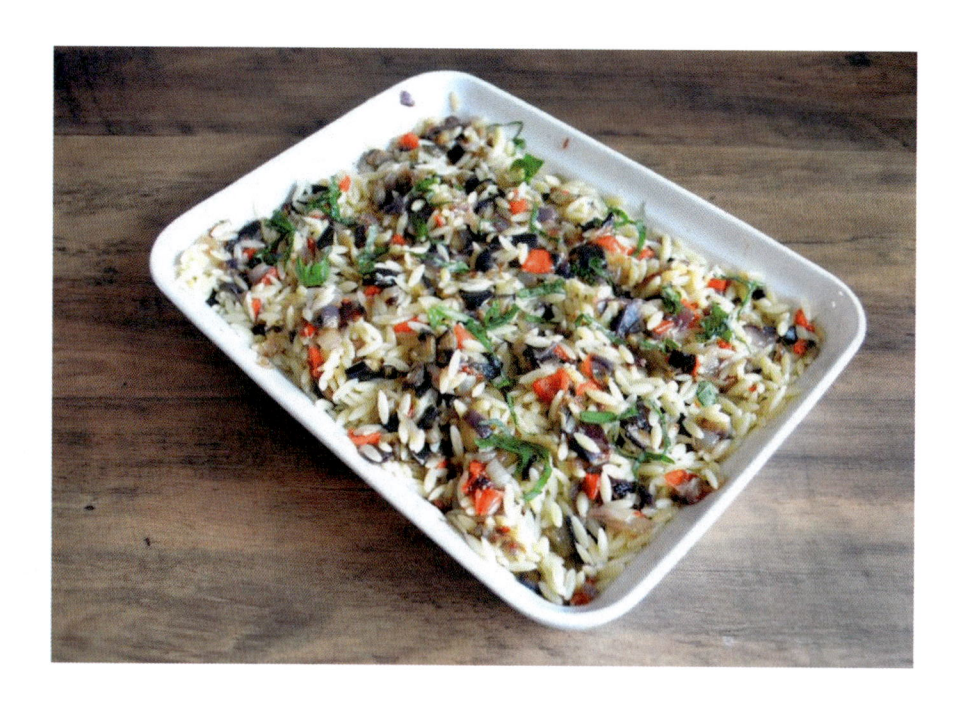

Method:

1. Set your oven to 200C/392F.

2. Dice all of your vegetables to a size that suits your child and place onto a baking tray with the black pepper and olive oil. Use your hands to mix well. Roast for 30-40 minutes, giving them a mix halfway through until the vegetables have slightly caramelised.

3. Meanwhile, cook the orzo according to the instructions on the packet (this usually takes about 10 minutes). Drain and place in a large serving or salad bowl.

4. Mix together the dressing ingredients (apart from the basil) in a small bowl or mug.

5. Mix the roasted vegetables into the cooked orzo and drizzle over the dressing.

6. Sprinkle over the basil leaves and serve! This can be eaten hot or as a cold salad.

-♦♦- -♦♦- -♦♦-

Time Boost – you may already have the roasted vegetable mix in the freezer if you have made it previously, so just defrost and mix in with cooked orzo! Alternatively, use a food processor to dice all of your vegetables.

Alternative Twist – you could try adding pieces of roast chicken, flaked salmon or for older children, pieces of sausage. If serving as a salad, add cubes of feta cheese (be careful, as this is too salty for babies). Adults could also add pine nuts or olives to their orzo.

BLACK BEANS AND PAPAYA

10 mins preparation
15 mins cooking
Serves 4

1 red onion, diced to a suitable size for your child
2 cloves of garlic, crushed
1/2 a glass of orange juice
A squeeze of lemon juice
1/2 a teaspoon of cayenne pepper
1 red pepper, diced or sliced to a suitable size for your child
1 papaya, diced
400g/large tin of black beans or adzuki beans (lentils also work well)
2 dessert spoons of fresh coriander, chopped (optional)
Olive oil

Method:

1. Heat the olive oil in a pan over a medium heat. Add the onion and garlic and fry until soft.
2. Add in all of the remaining ingredients except the beans and coriander. Mix well and cook for 5-10 minutes, adding a little more orange juice if the mixture is dry and starts sticking.
3. Throw in the beans and cook for another 5 minutes.
4. Sprinkle over the coriander and serve with rice or pieces of chunky bread!

-♦♦- -♦♦- -♦♦-

Alternative Twist - why not experiment with mango instead of the papaya? Or perhaps mix it in with rice and serve cold as a salad.

Storage – this can be frozen in portions for up to 2 months

CHICKEN SATAY

15 mins preparation (plus 2 hours or overnight for marinating)
15 mins cooking
Serves 4-6

650g mini chicken breast fillets (or cut chicken breasts into strips)
1 teaspoon of ground coriander
1 teaspoon of ground fennel seeds (optional)
1 ½ teaspoons of ground cumin
3 cloves of garlic, crushed
Juice of half a lime
1/4 of a cup/150ml thick coconut milk
2.5 cm of fresh ginger, peeled and finely grated
1 level teaspoon of sugar
1 teaspoon of tamarind paste (from most major supermarkets)
1 teaspoon of turmeric powder
1 teaspoon of oil

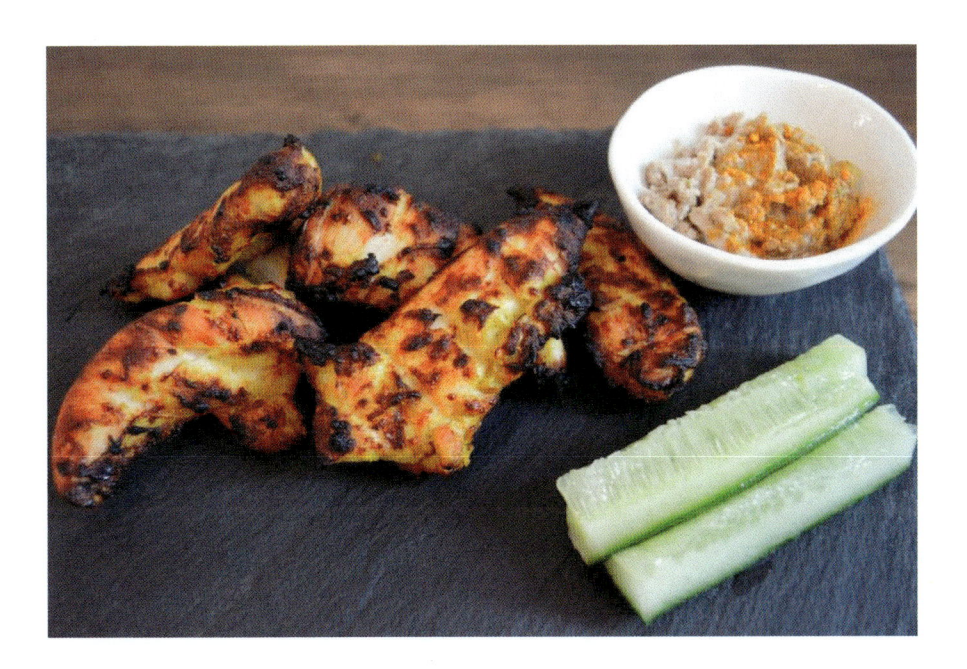

Method:

1. Roast the coriander, fennel and cumin briefly in a dry pan until aromatic.
2. Place the spices and the remaining ingredients into a large bowl to form a marinade and add the chicken.
3. Leave to marinate for at least 2 hours (overnight is best).
4. Set your grill to a medium heat and cook the chicken pieces for 5-7 minutes on each side until chargrilled.
5. Serve with peanut satay sauce and cucumber sticks!

-♦♦- -♦♦- -♦♦-

Storage - best served immediately but can be stored in the freezer for up to 2 months as an alternative to chicken nuggets!

Alternative Twist - put the chicken onto skewers and cook them on the barbecue or under the grill as a party snack. Try using strips of beef instead of chicken. You could also serve it in a tortilla wrap with fresh salad and a little sour cream!

Time Boost - place all of the marinade ingredients into a blender and blend until relatively smooth.

PEANUT SATAY SAUCE

10 mins preparation
10 mins cooking

2 teaspoons of ground coriander
1 teaspoon of ground cumin
1/2 a teaspoon of ground fennel seeds
1/2 a teaspoon of chilli powder
2 cloves of garlic, crushed
3 small shallots or 2 large spring onions, chopped
Juice of 1/2 a lime
2 heaped dessert spoons of 100% peanut butter
1 teaspoon of tamarind paste (from most major supermarkets)
3/4 of a cup/250 ml of thick coconut milk
1/4 of a cup/100 ml of water

Method:

1. Heat a little oil in a pan over a medium heat and add in the coriander, cumin, fennel, chilli, garlic, lime juice and shallots/spring onions. Fry for 3 minutes.
2. Add the peanut butter and slowly stir in the coconut milk.
3. Add the water and bring almost to the boil before turning down the heat and simmering until the oil starts to rise to the surface (5-10 mins).
4. Serve with chicken satay and cucumber sticks!

-♦♦- -♦♦- -♦♦-

Storage - this can be kept in the fridge for up to 3 days.

Alternative Twist - serve this with burgers, kebabs or meat skewers. You could also use it as a dip for crackers or breadsticks.

BEEF TAGINE

10 mins preparation
2 hours cooking
Serves 4

1 large onion, diced or sliced (depending on your baby's preference)
2 cloves of garlic, crushed
2.5 cm piece of ginger, peeled and finely grated
400g stewing beef, diced
400g (1 large tin) of chopped tomatoes
A small handful (or small 14g box) of raisins/sultanas (optional)
6 dried apricots, chopped
200g tinned chickpeas
1 large carrot, diced (optional)
200ml very low salt vegetable or beef stock (found in most major supermarkets or use the veg stock recipe at the beginning of the book)

<u>Spice Mix</u>
1 teaspoon of paprika
1 teaspoon of turmeric
1 teaspoon of ground cinnamon
1 teaspoon of ground coriander
1/2 a teaspoon of cayenne pepper
A pinch of black pepper

<u>Method</u>:

1. Set your oven to 200C/392F.

2. Heat some oil in a pan over a medium heat and fry the onion until translucent.

3. Add in the garlic and ginger and fry for 2 more mins.

4. Throw in the diced beef and fry until browned on all sides.

5. Add the spice mix and fry for 2 mins ensuring that the beef is well covered.

6. Add the tomatoes, chickpeas, carrot, apricots and raisins/sultanas and mix well.

7. Transfer the mixture to a casserole dish and pour in enough stock to just cover the mixture.

8. Mix the ingredients well and cook in the oven for 2 to 2 ½ hours, stirring halfway through. Add more water if needed or if you like more sauce.

9. Remove from the oven and add a little cornflour dissolved in cold water to the tagine if you like a thicker sauce.

10. Serve with rice, cous cous or bread!

-♦♦- -♦♦- -♦♦-

Time Boost – use a food processor to dice your onion and carrot. Prepare a large batch of the spice mix and store in an airtight container if you make this dish often so you can simply add it when needed.

Effort Boost – follow steps 2 to 5 then throw everything in a slow cooker along with the stock and leave to cook for a few hours.

Alternative Twist – try this recipe with lamb or for vegetarians try mixed root vegetables with beans etc.

Veggie Boost – add a handful or two of chopped spinach for added nutrients.

Storage – this can be frozen in portions for up to 2 months.

INDIAN SPICED RICE

5 mins preparation
10 mins cooking
Serves 3-4

1 cup white rice
2 cups boiling water
1 teaspoon of turmeric powder
1/2 a teaspoon of cinnamon powder
3 cloves (optional)
5 cardamom pods, squashed (so that the seeds inside can release their flavour)
A small handful of unsalted cashew nuts (optional - only for older children and adults although they do end up soft after the cooking process)

Method:

1. Put all of the ingredients into a pot and mix thoroughly.
2. Cover and leave to cook for 10 minutes.
3. Remove the cloves and cardamom and serve!

-♦♦- -♦♦- -♦♦-

Effort Boost - place all of the ingredients into a deep microwavable dish and put it into the microwave for 10-12 mins!

Alternative Twist - try using additional spices such as ½ a teaspoon of powdered ginger or a few saffron strands. You could also try making garlic rice or adding thinly sliced mushrooms to make mushroom rice. Additionally, you can even put in some sultanas or raisins (but check the temperature of these before serving as they can get really hot). For a sweet twist, try adding some desiccated coconut. This rice is delicious served with curry or roasted chicken/beef/lamb.

CARIBBEAN CHICKEN STEW

15 mins preparation (plus 2 hours or overnight for marinating)
30 mins cooking
Serves 4-6

650g chicken breast (or chicken thighs, de-boned)
Juice of 1 lime
5 spring onions, chopped
6 cloves of garlic, crushed
1 tablespoon of light soy sauce
1 large white onion, diced to a suitable size for your child
4 sprigs of thyme
3 tomatoes, diced to a suitable size for your child
1 dessert spoon of tomato puree
Boiling water

Method:

1. Mix all of the ingredients together (except the tomato puree) in a large bowl, making sure that the chicken is well covered. Leave to marinade for at least 2 hours (overnight is best).
2. Remove the chicken from the marinade and fry in a little oil over a medium heat until opaque.
3. Add in the marinade and the tomato puree, mixing well.
4. Top up the mixture with just enough boiling water to barely cover the chicken.
5. Simmer for 20-25 minutes, stirring occasionally until the sauce has thickened.
6. Remove the thyme sprigs and serve with plain white rice or rice and peas (recipe on the next page)!

-♦♦- -♦♦- -♦♦-

Storage – this can be kept in the fridge for 2 days or in the freezer for up to 2 months.

Effort Boost – you can also place all of the ingredients into a slow cooker and leave to simmer for a few hours.

Alternative Twist - if you like a thicker sauce, dissolve 1 dessert spoon of cornflour in a little cold water and add to the mix.

Veggie Boost – why not add vegetables to this or make a vegetable only version! Good vegetables to use are potatoes, carrots, green/broad beans and peas.

-♦♦- -♦♦- -♦- -♦♦- -♦♦-

RICE AND PEAS

10 mins preparation
20-25 mins cooking
Serves 4-6

400g/1 large tin red kidney beans (preserved in water)
3 fresh tomatoes, diced to a suitable size for your child
400g/1 large tin coconut milk
450g white rice
1 large onion, diced to a suitable size for your child
2 garlic cloves, crushed
1 very low salt vegetable stock cube (in most major supermarkets or use the vegetable stock recipe at the beginning of the book, alternatively skipping this is fine)
4 sprigs of thyme
1 tablespoon of butter

Method:

1. Drain the liquid from the beans into a measuring jug. Add the coconut milk and enough water to make 960ml.
2. Place the liquid into a large pot with the beans, onions, tomatoes, garlic, stock cube, thyme and butter. Bring it to a boil.
3. Add the rice and stir until it comes back to the boil.
4. Reduce the heat, cover and leave to cook for 20-25 minutes, stirring occasionally.
5. Remove the thyme sprigs and serve with Caribbean Chicken Stew!

-♦♦- -♦♦- -♦♦-

Alternative Twist - try adding other types of beans or lentils into the rice instead of the kidney beans. Mix in cooked chicken pieces and serve as a one pot dish. This is also delicious served with curry.

CRISPY SALMON WITH GINGER AND SPRING ONION

5 mins preparation
10-15 mins cooking
Serves 3

260g boneless salmon fillets (with skin)
2.5cm ginger, peeled and finely grated
2 large spring onions, sliced
2 teaspoons of sesame oil
Oil for frying

Method:

1. Heat a little oil in a pan and add the ginger.

2. Place the salmon on top, skin side down and fry for 3-5 minutes until the skin is crispy.

3. Turn over the salmon and fry the other side until cooked (about 3-5 minutes).

4. Sprinkle the spring onions over the top and drizzle in the sesame oil. Carry on frying until the salmon is crispy on both sides, but still tender to touch.

5. Serve with rice, boiled new potatoes or green beans!

-♦♦- -♦♦- -♦♦-

Alternative Twist – for adults and older children add a splash of soy sauce to enhance the flavour. Or why not try adding a little crushed garlic in with the ginger or even a small drizzle of sweet chilli sauce!

Effort Boost – you can also steam the fish, so place all of the ingredients into a steamer and leave to cook for 10-15 mins.

BEEF AND ONION PIE

15 mins preparation
20 mins cooking
Serves 4-6

500g lean minced beef
320g ready rolled puff pastry
300ml very low salt beef stock (available from most major supermarkets)
1 heaped dessert spoon of tomato puree
1 large/2 medium onions
1 large bay leaf
A large pinch of ground black pepper
A pinch of white pepper (optional)
1 tablespoon of plain flour
Milk for glazing

Method:

1. Set your oven too 200C/392F.

2. Quarter your onions and thinly slice them (or dice them, depending on your baby's preference).

3. Heat a little oil in a pan over a medium heat and fry the onions until they start to brown.

4. Add in the beef mince and tomato puree. Fry until the beef has browned.

5. Stir in the plain flour, ensuring everything is well mixed and cook for 1-2 mins.

6. Throw in the bay leaf, white and black peppers and gradually add in the beef stock until a gravy forms. Keep adding the stock until you reach your desired consistency.

7. Remove the bay leaf and pour the beef and onion mixture into an ovenproof dish.

8. Unroll the puff pastry and place it over the beef mixture. Cut off any excess pastry and use a fork to crimp around the edges.

9. If desired, make some leaves/animals/letters out of the pastry offcuts and place them on top of the pie.

10. Use a knife to make a few slits in the top of the pie to allow the steam to escape and use a pastry brush to generously baste the top of the pie with the milk.

11. Place the pie into the oven and bake for 20 mins until the top is golden and the gravy is bubbling.

12. Remove from the oven and serve with mashed potatoes and fresh veg!

-♦♦- -♦♦- -♦♦-

Alternative Twist - instead of putting the pastry over the top you could try making pasties! When doing this make a thicker gravy so that the pastry doesn't become soggy. Alternatively, blind bake some savoury shortcrust pastry before adding the filling and a top to make a more traditional pie. You could also try topping the mince mix with mashed potato to make cottage pie.

Veggie Boost - try adding some cooked diced carrot, lentils or mushroom to boost those nutrients! This dish is particularly delicious served with peas, broccoli or green beans.

Time Boost - use a food processor to chop your onions.

CHICKEN CURRY

10 mins preparation
20 mins cooking
Serves 4

400g chicken breast or thigh, diced

2 tablespoons medium curry powder (mild and hot are also good, depending on your baby's taste)

8 curry leaves (optional)

1 large white onion

2 large cloves of garlic, crushed

2cm ginger, peeled and finely grated

1 large potato, diced to a size to suit your baby

200g/small tin chickpeas

2 tablespoons coconut milk

1 dessert spoon of cornflour

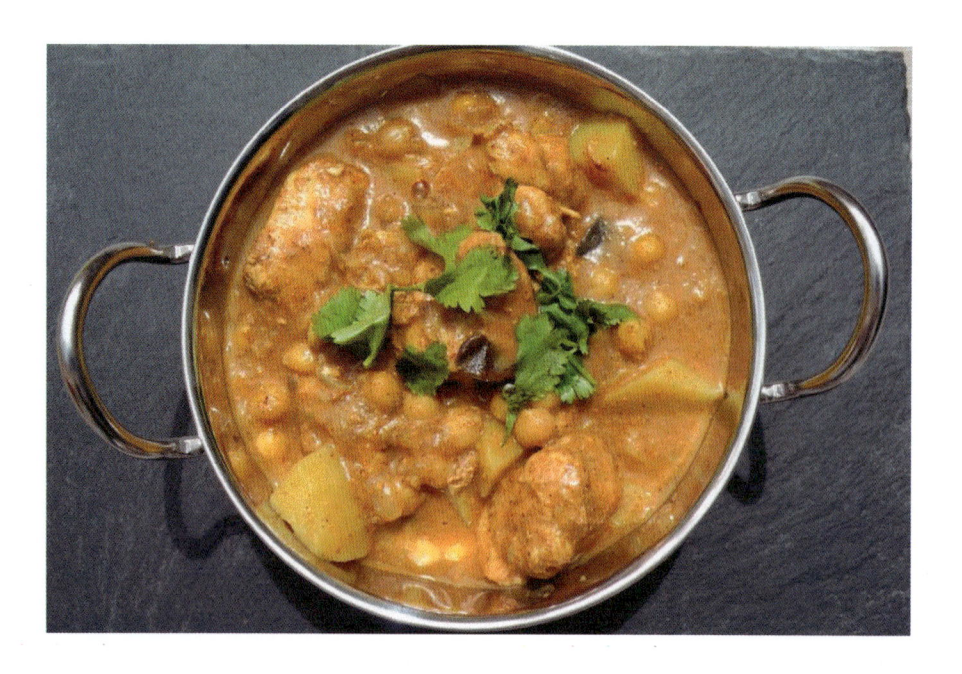

Method:

1. Dice the onion to a size that suits your baby. Heat a little oil in a pan over a medium heat, add the onion and fry until translucent.

2. Add in the crushed garlic, grated ginger, curry leaves and curry powder. Mix together and fry for 2 minutes.

3. Put the chicken in the pan and stir well. Fry until the chicken is opaque on all sides.

4. Add the potato, chickpeas and enough boiling water to just cover the chicken.

5. Cook for 15-20 minutes, stirring occasionally until the chicken is cooked and potatoes soft.

6. Lower the heat and add the coconut milk.

7. Dissolve the cornflour in a little cold water and add to the pan.

8. Stir and simmer for 5 minutes or until the sauce thickens.

9. Serve hot with delicious rice or naan bread!

-♦♦- -♦♦- -♦♦-

Alternative Twist - add sweet potato or butternut squash. Sprinkle some fresh coriander over the top to create another level of flavour.

Veggie Boost - add quartered cherry tomatoes, chopped spinach or diced carrots to make it extra delicious!

Effort Boost - use a food processor to dice your onion, garlic, ginger and even the potatoes!

Storage – this can be frozen in portions for up to 2 months.

SHEPHERD'S PIE

15 mins preparation
35 mins cooking
Serves 4

400g lean lamb mince
1 large onion, diced
1 large carrot, diced
1/2 a cup of peas
400ml very low salt vegetable stock
1 tablespoon of plain flour
1 tablespoon of tomato puree
1 teaspoon of dried rosemary or thyme
450g potatoes, peeled and diced
150ml milk
25g butter
A pinch of black pepper
50g grated cheddar cheese (optional)

Method:

1. Set your oven to 200C/392F.

2. Put the potatoes into a pot of boiling water and cook for 5-10 minutes until soft.

3. Meanwhile, put the carrots into a small pan of boiling water and cook until soft (or place the carrots in a bowl of boiling water and put it in the microwave for 3-5 mins).

4. While the carrots are cooking, put a little oil in a pan over a medium heat and add the onion. Fry until translucent.

5. Add the lamb mince and fry until browned.

6. Stir in the tomato puree, dried herbs and plain flour and fry for a couple of minutes.

7. Drain the carrots and add them into the mince mixture with the peas, giving everything a good mix.

8. Add the stock bit by bit until it thickens and you reach your preferred consistency.

9. Drain the potatoes and mash them with the milk, black pepper and butter.

10. Place the mince mixture into a large ovenproof dish and even it out before topping with the mashed potato.

11. Sprinkle with the grated cheese (if using) and place in the oven to cook for 20-30 mins.

12. Serve alone or with steamed broccoli or green beans!

-♦♦- -♦♦- -♦♦-

Time Boost – use a food processor to chop your onion and carrot.

Effort Boost – you can use ready made mashed potato from the supermarket, but be wary of the salt content.

Alternative Twist – try making a cottage pie by using beef instead of the lamb, low salt beef stock instead of vegetable stock and putting in a bay leaf instead of the rosemary/thyme.

Storage – you can follow steps 1 to 10 and freeze this in portions for up to 2 months.

CHINESE FRIED RICE

10 mins preparation
10 mins cooking
Serves 4

1 ½ cups of cooked white rice (1 day old is best, you can use freshly cooked rice but when fried it tends to go a little sticky/clumpy)

2 spring onions

1 large white onion

1 red pepper

100g peas

100g sweetcorn

1 large carrot, thinly sliced or use a peeler to make it into ribbons (to a size your baby can manage)

4 eggs, beaten

Oil for frying

1 dessert spoon of sesame oil

1 teaspoon of light soy sauce

Method:

1. Heat a little oil in a pan over a medium heat and add in the egg. Scramble and set aside once cooked.

2. Heat a little more oil in the pan and add in the white onion and fry until golden.

3. Add the remaining vegetables and fry for 3-4 minutes until they have softened a little.

4. Throw in the rice and break it up a little while mixing it in with all of the vegetables.

5. Drizzle the sesame oil and soy sauce over the rice (this will also help to separate the rice grains). Mix well.

6. Add the egg back into the pan and throw in the spring onion. Fry for 2 minutes until the egg has reheated.

7. Serve!

-♦♦- -♦♦- -♦♦-

Alternative Twist - add pieces of chopped up ham, sausage or bacon (be careful of the salt content when doing this) or even chicken or seafood! Try using other vegetables such as baby corn, broccoli etc.

Time Boost - I often use 1 cup of frozen mixed veg from the supermarket instead of the separate peas, carrot and sweetcorn! It defrosts very quickly in the pan and saves a lot of effort!

Effort Boost - use a food processor to chop up your onion and red pepper!

SINGAPORE NOODLES

20 mins preparation
10 mins cooking
Serves 4

250g dried rice vermicelli noodles
1 large white onion
1 large red pepper
2 spring onions
2.5cm fresh ginger
1 heaped dessert spoon of mild curry powder
1/2 a teaspoon of chilli powder (or more, depending on your baby, to taste)
1 teaspoon of turmeric powder
1 tablespoon of soy sauce

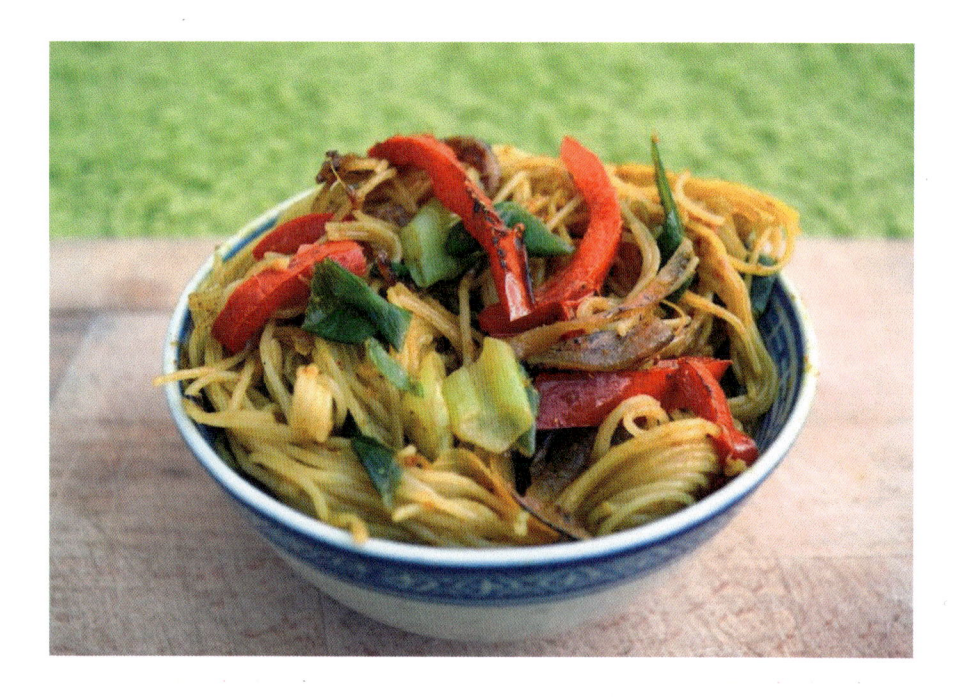

Method:

1. Soak the rice vermicelli noodles in a large bowl of cold water for 20 minutes until soft.

2. Meanwhile, chop the spring onions, slice the onion and pepper (to a size that your child can manage) and peel and finely grate the ginger.

3. Fry the onion in a little oil over a medium to high heat until golden (or even better, a bit charred).

4. Add the ginger and fry for 2 minutes.

5. Throw in the pepper, mix well and fry for 3 minutes.

6. Drain the noodles and add them to the pan.

7. Drizzle over the soy sauce and sprinkle over the curry powder. Give it a good mix and fry for 5 minutes, adding splashes of water if the mixture looks too dry.

7. Serve!

-♦♦- -♦♦- -♦♦-

Effort Boost - you can buy ready soaked/cooked rice vermicelli noodles from most major supermarkets so can just throw them in when needed!

Alternative Twist - add in cooked shredded chicken, beef and/or beansprouts when you put in the pepper.

Time Boost - use a food processor to chop up your onion, pepper and spring onions.

PASTA BAKE

15 mins preparation
20 mins cooking
Serves 4

200g pasta (fusilli or farfalle are good as they hold the sauce)

500g passata (you can buy 99% tomato passata which has a lower salt content)

1 large onion

2 cloves of garlic, crushed

1/3 of a teaspoon of cayenne pepper

250g ricotta

100g fresh spinach

1/3 of a teaspoon/pinch of nutmeg (optional)

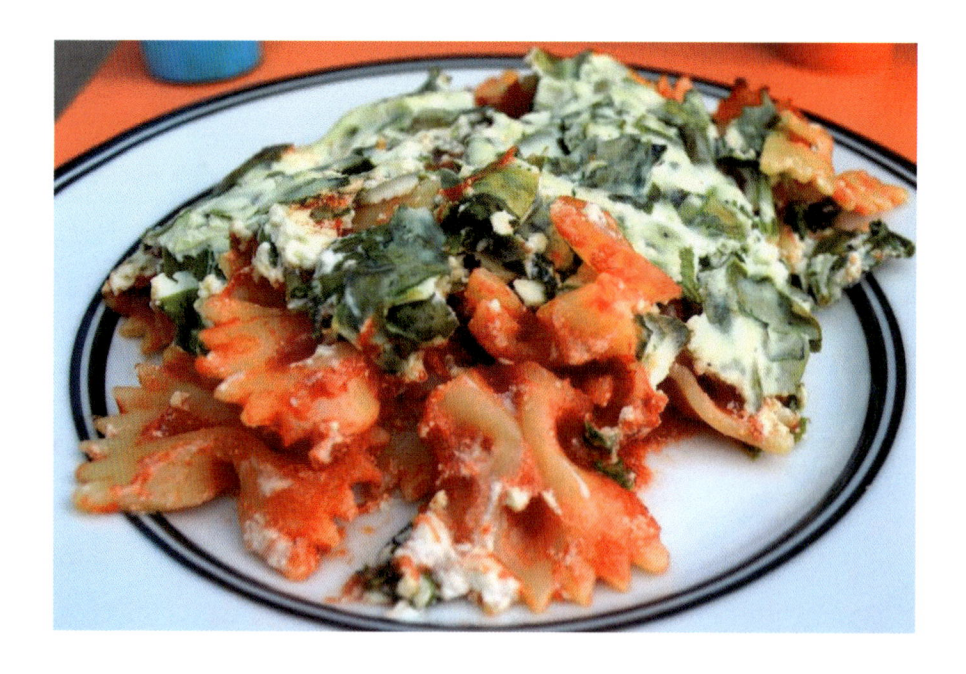

Method:

1. Preheat your oven too 200C/392F.

2. Put the pasta in a pot of boiling water and cook for 10 minutes.

3. Meanwhile, dice the onion and place it in a large pot with the garlic and fry until golden.

4. Add in the passata and cayenne pepper. Allow to simmer for 5-10 mins.

5. While the sauce is cooking, rinse and chop the spinach.

6. Place the ricotta into a pan and add the spinach. Stir until the spinach starts to wilt and the ricotta becomes smooth.

7. Add the nutmeg (if using) to the ricotta mixture and stir well.

8. Drain the pasta and mix it into the passata sauce.

9. Take an oven dish and line the bottom of it with the pasta.

10. Layer the spinach and ricotta mixture over the top of the pasta.

11. Cook in the oven for 15-20 minutes.

12. Serve!

-♦♦- -♦♦- -♦♦-

Alternative Twist - you can add beef mince, meatballs, sausage (watch out for the salt content) or even tuna to this dish - if so, use 250g more passata to create more sauce.

Vegetable Boost - try adding chopped peppers, mushrooms (grated for babies), grated carrot or even cooked butternut squash!

Effort Boost - use a food processor to chop your onion and garlic. You can also use it to chop the spinach and mix it with the ricotta/nutmeg at the same time.

SUNDRIED TOMATO RISOTTO

5 mins preparation
25 mins cooking
Serves 4

250g Arborio risotto rice

700ml very low salt vegetable or chicken stock (or use the recipe at the beginning of the book)

1 large white onion

280g jar of sundried tomatoes (you only need 6-8 sundried tomatoes depending on how strong you want your risotto)

1 clove of garlic, crushed

1 teaspoon of tomato puree

A pinch of black pepper

1 tablespoon of olive oil (or even better, use the olive oil from the jar of sundried tomatoes for an extra flavour boost!)

200g chopped spinach (optional)

30g grated mozzarella

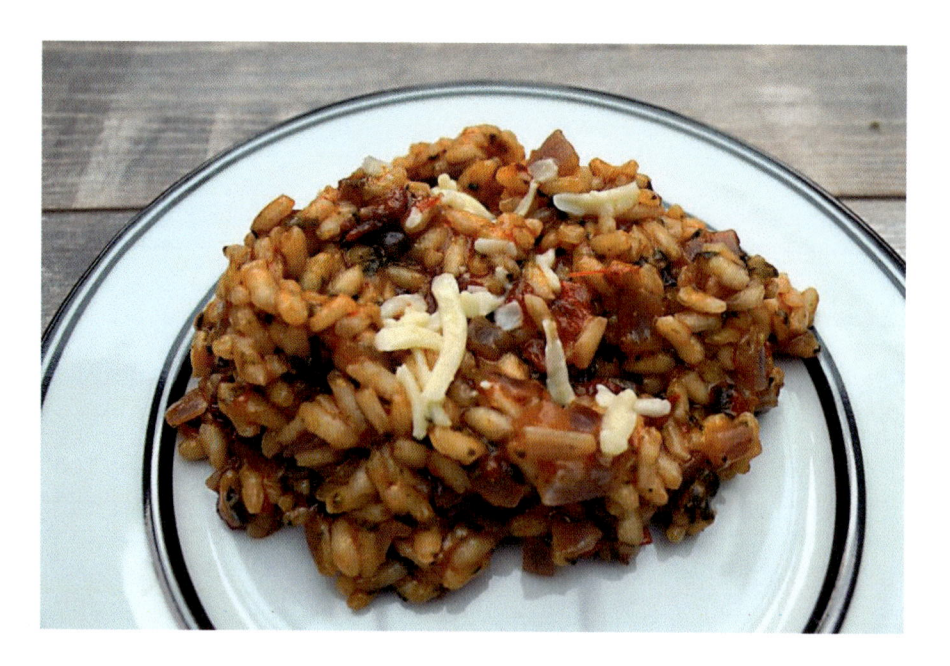

Method:

1. Take 6-8 sundried tomatoes from the jar and chop them into smaller pieces. Set them aside.

2. Use one tablespoon of olive oil from the jar of sundried tomatoes and heat it in a pan over a medium heat. Add the onions and fry until translucent.

2. Add the garlic, sundried tomatoes, black pepper and tomato puree into the pan and fry for 2-3 mins until the garlic has cooked.

3. Throw in the risotto rice and fry for another 3 mins, ensuring the rice is well covered with the mixture.

4. Add in one ladleful of the stock and stir until all of the stock has been absorbed. Repeat this process until you have used up all of the stock (about 20 mins).

5. Stir in the chopped spinach (if using) and cook until it has wilted (2 mins).

6. Turn off the heat and put a lid on the pan. Leave for 5 mins for the rice to swell.

7. Sprinkle over the mozzarella and serve!

-♦♦- -♦♦- -♦♦-

Alternative Twist - add in some cooked prawns or shellfish (beware of allergies) to make a seafood risotto! You could try the same method using peas or mushroom instead of the sundried tomatoes (also leave out the tomato puree). You can use grated parmesan instead of the mozzarella, but be wary of the salt content!

Time Boost - use kitchen scissors to cut your sundried tomatoes. You can also use a food processor to chop your onion, garlic, sundried tomatoes and spinach.

Effort Boost - you can also cook this in the oven! Set your oven to 200C/392F. Prepare steps 1 to 3 above, then put all of the ingredients in an ovenproof dish along with the stock. Mix it all well, cover and place in the oven for 20-30 minutes. Remove the risotto once the rice is cooked and sprinkle the mozzarella over the top.

-♦♦- SNACKS -♦♦-

CARROT AND OAT SOFTIE BISCUITS

15 mins preparation
10 mins cooking
Makes 16-20 biscuits

85-95g (or 1 large) carrot, finely grated

115g butter, softened

70g soft light brown sugar

25g desiccated coconut

25g rolled porridge oats

150g self raising flour

1 large egg

½ a teaspoon of vanilla extract

½ a teaspoon of ground cinnamon

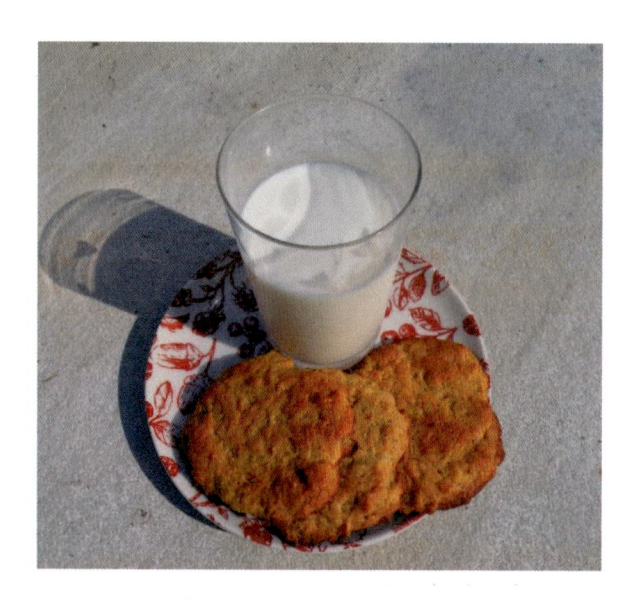

Method:

1. Set your oven to 190C/375F.
2. Take a large mixing bowl and beat the butter and sugar together until pale and creamy.
3. Beat in the egg and vanilla extract until smooth.
4. Sift in the flour and cinnamon and mix with a metal spoon.
5. Add the grated carrot, coconut and oats. Mix well.
6. Place heaped teaspoonfuls of the mixture onto a non-stick baking tray or sheet. Flatten each biscuit with the back of the spoon.
7. Bake in the oven for 10-15 minutes or until golden.
8. Remove from the oven and leave to cool for 2-3 minutes on the tray before transferring to a wire cooling rack to cool completely.
9. Serve!

-♦♦- -♦♦- -♦♦-

Alternative Twist - why not add some dried fruit such as raisins or for older children, chopped mixed nuts? For crispy biscuits, substitute the self raising flour for plain flour.

Storage – store in an airtight container for up to 3 days.

CANDIED ORANGE CUPCAKES

15 mins preparation
15 mins cooking
Makes 12 cupcakes

100g butter, softened
50g sugar
1 medium egg
100g self raising flour, sifted
½ a teaspoon of baking powder
50g candied peel

Method:

1. Set your oven to 180C/356F.
2. Place the butter and sugar into a large mixing bowl and beat until light and fluffy.
3. Add the egg and mix well.
4. Slowly add in the flour and baking powder, stirring in a figure of eight motion.
5. Add in the candied peel and continue mixing carefully to ensure you don't knock out too much air.
6. Line a cupcake tin with cupcake cases and fill each case with the cupcake mixture.
7. Bake for 12-15 minutes or until golden.
8. Remove from the oven and allow to cool on a wire rack before serving.

-♦♦- -♦♦- -♦♦-

Storage – The cupcakes can be kept in an airtight container for a couple of days. Alternatively, they can be frozen for up to 6 weeks.

Alternative Twist – try using different kinds of dried fruit (or even a little bit of stewed fruit) in the mixture instead of the candied peel! For a really decadent treat, make a cream cheese frosting by using mascarpone with a little bit of vanilla essence or cinnamon.

VEGETABLE TARTLETS

20 mins preparation
20-30 mins cooking time
Makes 12-16 tartlets

1 courgette

1 small aubergine

1 red onion

1 red pepper, deseeded

1 clove of garlic, crushed

A pinch of black pepper

1 tablespoon of olive oil

250g ricotta cheese

320g ready rolled puff pastry

Milk or melted butter for basting

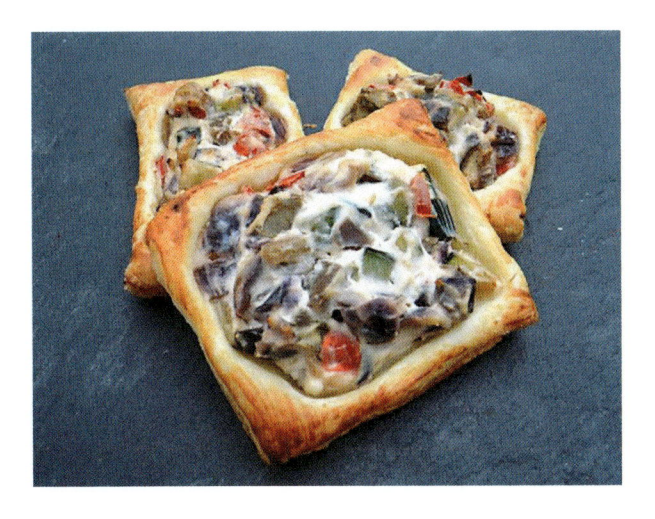

Method:

1. Set your oven to 220C/428F.
2. Dice all of the vegetables to a size that your child can manage.
3. Put the olive oil into a pan over a medium heat and fry the onion until softened.
4. Add the garlic and fry for 2 minutes.

5. Add the remaining vegetables and fry until softened and slightly caramelised (10-15 mins). Season with the black pepper. Set aside to cool a little.
6. Unwrap your puff pasty and spread it out on a flat, lightly floured surface.
7. Cut the pastry into 12-16 squares, depending on what size you would like your tartlets (alternatively, use a biscuit cutter to cut out circles to your desired size).
8. Place the ricotta into a bowl and add the roasted vegetable mix and black pepper. Mix well.
9. Spoon heaped teaspoonfuls of the ricotta mixture into the centre of each pastry square/disc making sure there is still a small ring of pastry around the outside.
10. Place the tartlets onto a lightly greased baking tray or sheet. Brush a little butter or milk around the edges of each tartlet.
11. Bake for 15-20 minutes until the ricotta has browned slightly and the pasty is golden and puffy.
12. Serve immediately or once cool as a delicious snack!

-♦♦- -♦♦- -♦♦-

Storage – the tartlets can be kept in an airtight container in the fridge for 2 days or in the freezer for up to 6 weeks.

Time Boost – for a quick vegetable mix, dice all of the vegetables in a food processor.

Effort Boost – the roasted vegetable mix is great to use in this recipe! (The recipe for this is at the beginning of the book) Simply mix it into the ricotta and season with black pepper.

Alternative Twist – make larger tarts so that you have one each for lunch, or even make a puff pasty pizza by simply unrolling the pasty and using it at its full size. You can mix any leftover ricotta mix into cooked pasta to create a delicious meal or pasta salad. For a truly decadent twist you can add smoked salmon on top of the tartlets (but beware of the salt content if giving to babies).

GUACAMOLE WITH TORTILLA CHIPS

10 mins preparation
10 mins cooking
Serves 4

1 large, very ripe avocado

A pinch of white pepper

1 sprig of coriander (optional), chopped

Juice of ½ a lime

1/2 a clove of garlic, crushed

4-5 tortilla wraps

1 teaspoon of smoked paprika

Olive oil

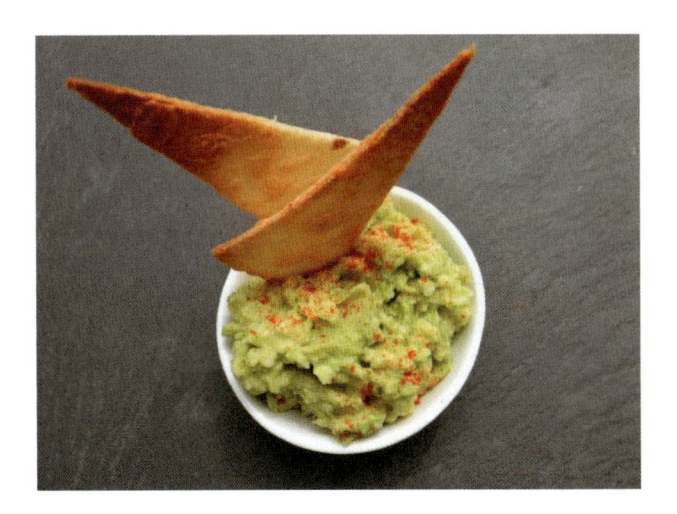

Method:

1. Set your oven to 200C/392F.

2. Brush the tortilla wraps lightly on each side in a little olive oil before cutting them into triangles.

3. Spread the tortilla chips out evenly on a baking tray and put them in the oven to bake until crispy (about 5 minutes).

4. Meanwhile, cut the avocado in half, discard the stone and remove the flesh.

5. Place the avocado in a bowl and mash with a fork.

6. Add the lime juice, coriander, garlic and white pepper and mix thoroughly.

7. Check on your tortilla chips and remove them from the oven if crispy. Sprinkle over the smoked paprika and serve!

-♦♦- -♦♦- -♦♦-

Alternative Twist – add some chopped tomato, sweetcorn or peppers into your guacamole to create other flavours. For a different flavour you could buy flavoured tortilla wraps with herbs already added. To make them more fun you could also use a cookie cutter to make different shaped tortilla chips! You could even try making pitta chips by cutting up and toasting pitta bread.

Time Boost – place the guacamole ingredients into a blender or use a hand held blender and mix until you reach your desired consistency!

Storage – you can store the tortilla chips in an airtight container for up to 3 days. The guacamole is best eaten on the same day that it is prepared.

KALE CRISPS

5 mins preparation
10 mins cooking

100g of kale, chopped
2 teaspoons of oil

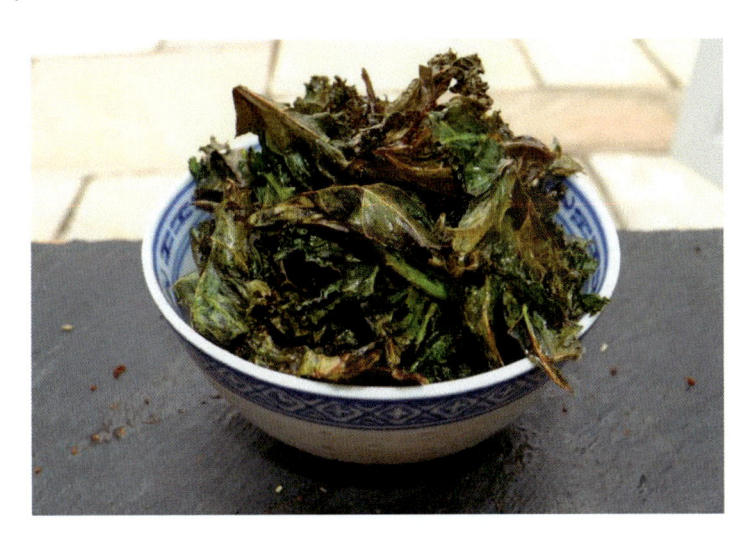

Method:

1. Set your oven to 200C/392F.
2. Wash and drain the kale. Shake off the excess water and place it onto a small baking tray.
3. Drizzle the oil over the top and using your hands toss the kale well in the oil.
4. Place the tray into the oven for 10 minutes.
5. Remove from the oven and enjoy your crunchy and healthy kale crisps!

-♦♦- -♦♦- -♦♦-

Alternative Twist - try using different vegetables to make crisps! All you need is to use a vegetable peeler to cut your vegetables into ribbons - good ones to try are potatoes/sweet potatoes, carrots, spinach, courgettes.

Storage – these are best served immediately but can be stored in an airtight container for a couple of days.

BREAD ROLL PIZZAS

5 mins preparation
10 mins cooking

Finger Rolls (or other bread rolls/paninis/tortillas or pittas will do)
Tomato Puree
Cheese
A pinch of Italian mixed herbs/oregano/basil

Method:

1. Set your oven to 200C/392F.

2. Halve the finger roll as if you are making a sandwich.

3. Spread the tomato puree onto each half and sprinkle the herbs on top.

4. Add sliced or grated cheese on top.

5. Bake in the oven for 10 mins or until the cheese has melted.

6. Serve as a delicious snack or simple lunch!

-♦♦- -♦♦- -♦♦-

Alternative Twist - try using different types of cheese (but be wary of the salt content!). Good ones to use are emmental, mozzarella or smoked cheese. You could also try adding pre-cooked/leftover chicken or even tinned tuna (preserved in spring water, not brine). Alternatively, perhaps use red or green pesto instead of the tomato puree.

Veggie Boost - add some sweetcorn, sliced onions or peppers on top!

-♦♦- DRINKS -♦♦-

Ideally, babies and toddlers should be offered plain water with meals, but here are a few ideas for a special treat or those times when they just don't want to drink!

-♦♦- -♦♦- -♦- -♦♦- -♦♦-

CITRUS WATER

- 1 wedge or 1 thick slice of lemon/lime/orange
- 1 glass/½ a pint of cool water (still or sparkling)

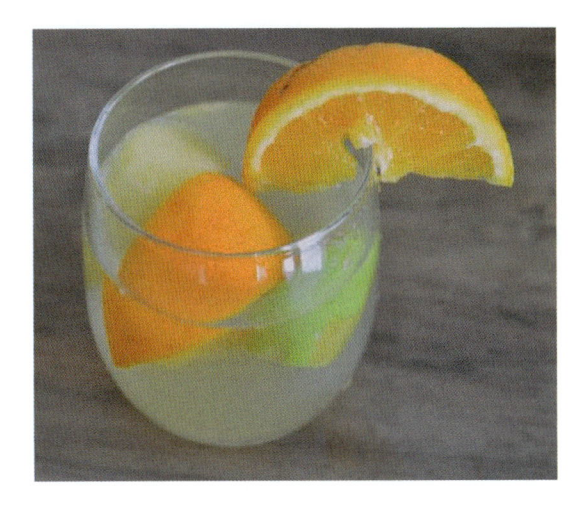

Method:

1. Squeeze the juice from the wedge or slice of fruit into a tumbler/plastic cup.

2. Add the water and give it a stir.

3. Serve!

Alternative Twist – why not try other fruits in this! How about some grapefruit, mushed up peaches/nectarines or melon? Or perhaps mix several fruits in a whole jug of water!

KIDDIE PIÑA COLADA

- 50g fresh pineapple
- 1 tablespoon of coconut milk
- ½ a medium banana
- 200ml cool water
- Edible flowers (such as pansies, nasturtiums or violas) or mint leaves – optional

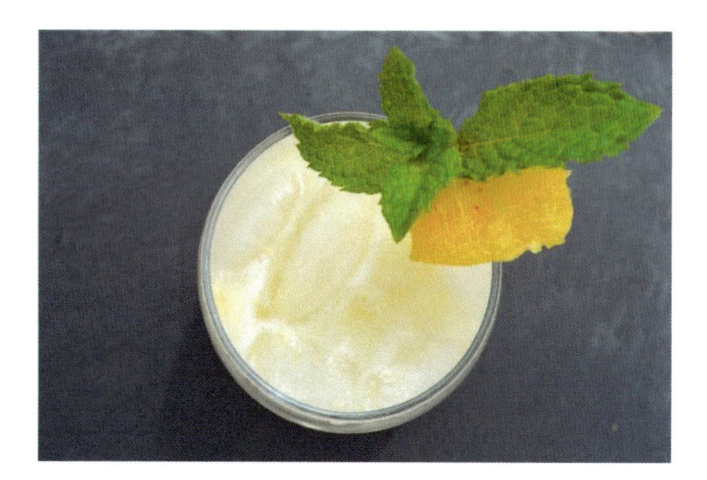

Method:

1. Put all of the ingredients into a blender and blend until smooth.

2. Decorate with the rinsed edible flowers or mint leaves (if using them).

3. Serve cold as a refreshing drink!

BERRY COOLER

- 1 small handful of berries of your choice (strawberries, blueberries, raspberries and blackberries are good, or even a mixture of all of them!)
- 1 Jug/1 litre of cool water (still or sparkling)

Method:

1. Place the berries into a bowl and squash lightly with a fork.

2. Put them into the jug and add the water.

3. Give it all a stir and serve!

Alternative Twist – add a sprig of mint or rosemary to this to give it a more interesting flavour! You could also add a dessert spoon of stewed apple.

-♦♦- -♦♦- -♦- -♦♦- -♦♦-

APPLE, MINT AND LIME COOLER

10 mins preparation
Serves 4-6

900ml cool water (still or sparkling)
100ml apple juice (fresh is preferable)
1 Lime
Large sprig of mint

Method:

1. Put the water into a large jug and add the apple juice and juice of ½ the lime.

2. Tear the leaves off the mint sprig and either roll in your hands or rip into small pieces. Add to the water and juice mix.

3. Stir together and serve with wedges made from the remainder of the lime.

Alternative Twist - Try adding some crushed raspberries, cucumber slices or even a sprig of rosemary in the mix!

WEANING DIARY

Date	Food(s)	Like	Unsure	Refuse

BABY-LED WEANING FOR BUSY PARENTS

Date	Food(s)	Like	Unsure	Refuse

OLIVIA WITHALL

Date	Food(s)	Like	Unsure	Refuse

-♦- DAILY MENU -♦-

Date:

Today I have eaten…

When	Breakfast	Snack	Lunch	Snack	Dinner
What					
All					
½					
¼					
None					

Date:

Today I have eaten…

When	Breakfast	Snack	Lunch	Snack	Dinner
What					
All					
½					
¼					
None					

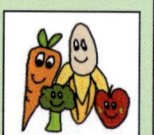

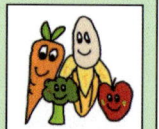

Date:

Today I have eaten…

When	Breakfast	Snack	Lunch	Snack	Dinner
What					
All					
½					
¼					
None					

Date:

Today I have eaten…

When	Breakfast	Snack	Lunch	Snack	Dinner
What					
All					
½					
¼					
None					

-♦♦- ACE AND EVE'S FOOD DIARY -♦♦-

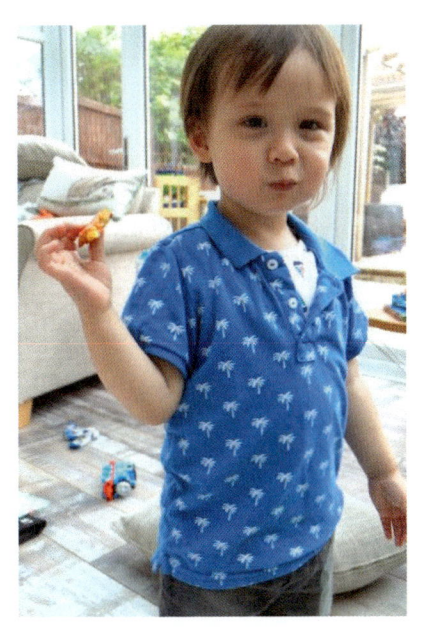

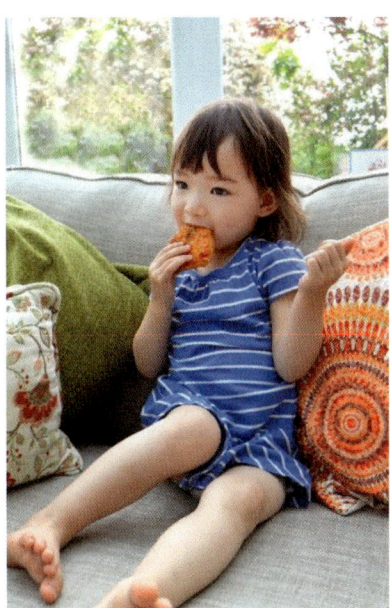

Date	Food	ACE	EVE
29 March	Roasted Carrot	Liked	Loved
	Roasted Potato	Refused	Liked
	Roasted Sweet Potato	Liked	Liked
	Roasted Broccoli	Refused	Refused
30 March	Rice Cake	Liked	Liked
31 March	Hard Boiled Egg	Liked	Liked
	Orange	Loved	Loved
1 April	Porridge with stewed apple	Liked	Liked
	Greek Yoghurt	Loved	Liked
	Houmous	Liked	Refused
	Mango	Liked	Loved
	Giant fusilli pasta with tomato and garlic sauce	Loved	Liked

Date	Food	ACE	EVE
2 April	Spring onion omelette	Loved	Refused
	Rice Cake	Loved	Loved
	Orange	Loved	Loved
3 April	Pancake with stewed apple	Loved	Loved
	Greek Yoghurt	Loved	Loved
	Mango	Loved	Loved
4 April	Toast with cashew nut butter	Liked	Loved
	Strawberries	Refused	Liked
	Tenderstem Broccoli	Liked	Liked
5 April	Chilli con carne with rice	Liked	Loved
	Orange	Loved	Loved
6 April	Strawberry	Loved	Liked
	Greek Yoghurt	Loved	Loved
	Jaffa Orange	Loved	Loved
	Rice Cake	Liked	Liked
7 April	Toast with unsalted butter	Loved	Loved
	Mango	Liked	Refused
	Greek Yoghurt	Loved	Loved
	Blueberries	Liked	Loved
	Rice Cake	Loved	Loved
8 April	Toast with almond butter	Liked	Liked
	Scrambled Egg	Loved	Liked
	Papaya	Loved	Liked
	Rice Cake	Liked	Liked
9 April	Porridge with stewed pear	Loved	Loved
	Jaffa Orange	Loved	Loved
	Toast with cashew nut butter	Liked	Liked

BABY-LED WEANING FOR BUSY PARENTS

Date	Food	ACE	EVE
	Pear	Liked	Liked
10 April	Porridge with stewed apple	Loved	Loved
	Homemade pizza (tomato, garlic and ricotta)	Loved	Liked
	Papaya	Loved	Liked
11 April	Toast with cashew nut butter	Loved	Liked
	Greek yoghurt	Loved	Loved
	Cucumber	Loved	Refused
	Banana	Refused	Loved
12 April	Eggy bread	Loved	Liked
	Chicken cooked in sesame oil	Loved	Loved
	Baby sweetcorn	Loved	Loved
13 April	Porridge with stewed pear	Liked	Liked
	Watermelon	Loved	Loved
	Cucumber	Loved	Loved
	Nectarine	Loved	Liked
14 April	Toast with unsalted butter	Liked	Refused
	Greek yoghurt with stewed apple	Loved	Loved
	Houmous	Refused	Liked
	Kiwi Fruit	Refused	Refused
	Cantaloupe Melon	Liked	Liked
15 April	Rice Cake	Liked	Liked
	Banana	Liked	Refused
	Mushroom Risotto (with ricotta)	Loved	Loved
16 April	Greek yoghurt with stewed nectarine	Loved	Loved
	Cannelloni with tomato, carrot, black pepper and paprika sauce	Loved	Loved
	Strawberries	Loved	Loved

OLIVIA WITHALL

Date	Food	ACE	EVE
17 April	Porridge with stewed apple	Loved	Loved
	Salmon (fried in ginger and sesame oil)	Loved	Refused
	Cucumber	Loved	Loved
	Mango	Loved	Loved
18 April	Pikelet with cashew nut butter	Loved	Loved
	Egg mayonnaise (only a bit of mayo because of salt)	Liked	Loved
19 April	Pikelet with unsalted butter	Liked	Liked
	Gnocchi with mascarpone, garlic, leek and mushroom sauce	Loved	Loved
	Mango	Loved	Loved
20 April	Greek yoghurt with stewed apple	Loved	Loved
	Fried chicken (cornflour/sesame oil)	Loved	Refused
	Cucumber	Loved	Loved
21 April	Pikelet with almond butter	Loved	Loved
	Rice cake	Liked	Liked
	Houmous	Liked	Liked
	Ratatouille with homemade bread rolls	Loved	Loved
22 April	Homemade bread roll	Loved	Loved
	Ratatouille	Loved	Loved
	Orzo pasta	Loved	Loved
	Watermelon	Loved	Loved

INDEX

A

Apple, Mint and Lime Cooler · 75

B

Bean Chilli · 28
Beef and Onion Pie · 50
Beef Tagine · 44
Berry Cooler · 75
Black Beans and Papaya · 40
Bread Roll Pizzas · 72

C

Candied Orange Cupcakes · 66
Caribbean Chicken Stew · 47, 48
Carrot and Oat Softie Biscuits · 64
Cauliflower and Broccoli Cheese · 30
Chicken Curry · 52
Chicken Satay · 41
Chinese Fried Rice · 56
Citrus Water · 73
Crispy Salmon with Ginger and Spring Onion · 49

E

Egg and Tomato Scrumble · 24

F

Food for Teething · 8

G

Guacamole with Tortilla Chips · 69

H

Houmous · 17

I

Indian Spiced Rice · 46

K

Kale Crisps · 71
Kiddie Pina Colada · 74

L

Lentil Daal · 26

P

Paella · 34
Pasta Bake · 60
Pasta Sauce · 11
Peanut Satay Sauce · 43
Porridge · 16
Potato Wedges · 32

R

Ratatouille · 23
Rice and Peas · 48
Rice Pudding · 21
Roasted Vegetable Mix · 13
Roasted Vegetable Orzo · 38

S

Salt · 4
Shepherd's Pie · 54
Singapore Noodles · 58
Stewed Fruit · 9

Sugar · 4
Sundried Tomato Butter · 19
Sundried Tomato Risotto · 62
Sweetcorn Fritters · 35

V

Vegetable Stock · 10
Vegetable Tartlets · 67

W

Whipped Yoghurt Mousse · 18
White Sauce · 12

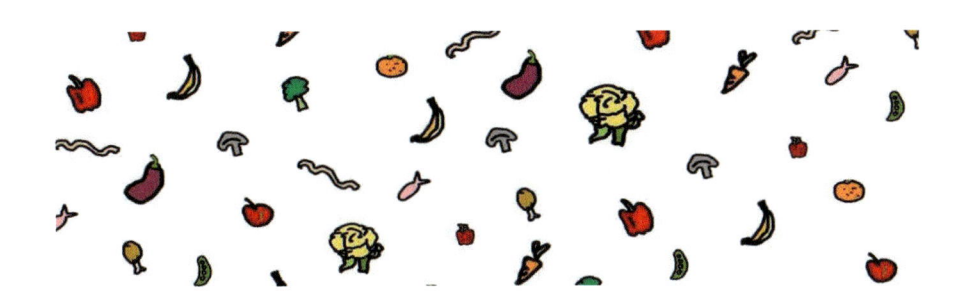

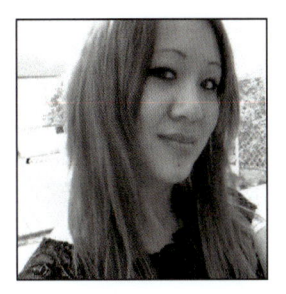

ABOUT THE AUTHOR

Olivia Withall always had a love for cooking and tasting new cuisines when travelling abroad with her husband, but became even more passionate about using fresh ingredients to prepare nutritious food when weaning her boy/girl twins, Ace and Eve. Olivia was born in the UK to Malaysian parents and has a BA (Hons) degree in English Literature from Queen Mary, University of London. She went on to enjoy a successful career as a Legal PA at several international law firms before eventually starting her own hand-crafted homeware business and furthering her culinary skills. Olivia lives in Essex, UK with the twins and her husband, James.

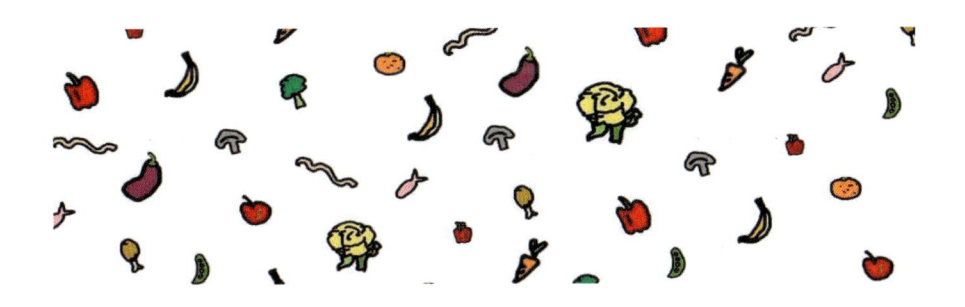

OLIVIA WITHALL

Printed in Great Britain
by Amazon